I0457814

ALZHEIMER'S DISEASE

LIVING WITH JOHN, CARING FOR A LOVE ONE

"The Long Lonely Road" A True Story of
Love, Hope and Triumph Over Personal Tragedy

SECOND EDITION - LARGE PRINT

NELLIE KIDD-MADISON

Copyright 2025 by Nellie Kidd-Madison

ISBN: 978-1-969422-44-7 (Paperback)
      978-1-969422-63-8 (Hardback)
      978-1-969422-45-4 (Ebook)

All rights reserved. No part of this book may be reproduced, distributed or transmitted in any form or by any means, including photocopying, recording or other electronic or mechanical methods, without the prior written permission of the publisher, except in the case brief quotations embodied in critical reviews and other noncommercial uses permitted by copyright law.

The views expressed in this book are solely those of the author and do not necessarily reflect the views of the publisher, and the publisher hereby disclaims any responsibility of them.

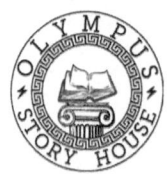

Olympus Story House
www.olympusstoryhouse.com

CONTENTS

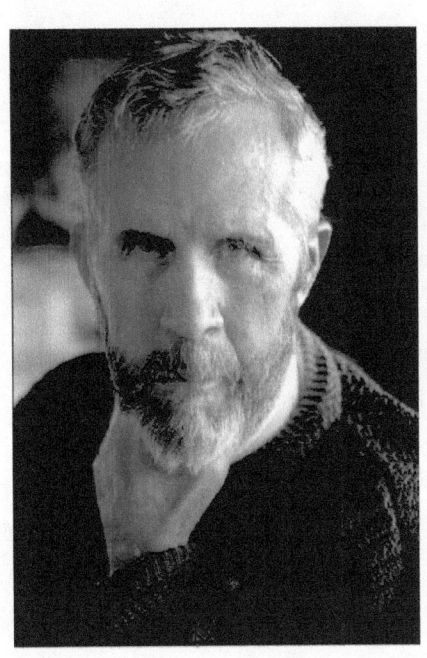

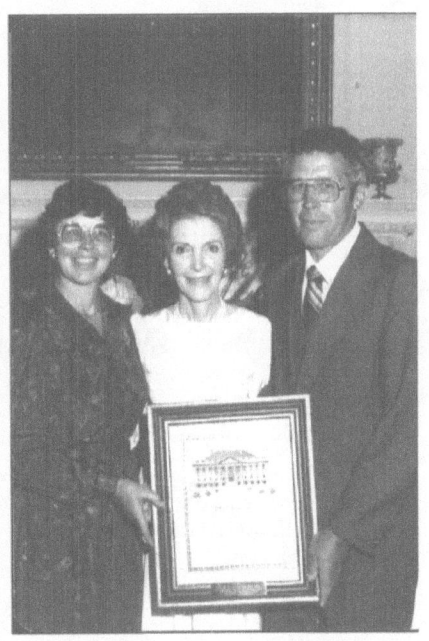

John Madison
1933-2002
69 years old

John and Nellie with
Nancy Reagan
1983-White House
Great American Family
One of Nine in Nation

I would like to dedicate this book to our four children, Valerie, Mark, Scott, and Kent; who were guided to adulthood by a loving father. Also to their nine children, who really never got to enjoy their grandfather's true affectionate personality. He would have had fun spoiling them!

ACKNOWLEDGEMENTS

I would like to thank friends and family who have helped to edit this book. Writing my story was surprisingly easy but to make it understandable has been the hard work. A writer knows what he or she is trying to say but to be sure that the reader understands the written thought is an entirely different matter. People who have not read my book believe that writing my story must have helped me mentally and suggest I start a second book. People who have read the book seem to understand helping others is what my book is all about and believe me when I say; "I have said it all!"

PREFACE

My husband, John Madison has Alzheimer's disease and I am Nellie, his wife and caregiver. We met forty-seven years ago at Oregon State College on a blind date. He was majoring in Agriculture while I was studying Home Economics. It was love at first sight for both or us and we have had an ideal marriage.

John was a true dirt farmer, loving his daily life of working the soil in the area of the Oregon Trail that crosses the width of our ranch. Raising grain and hay to feed his cowherd gave him a reason to rise early and greet, "the best part of the day." John never wanted to be anything else but a farmer. He has won almost every award available for conservation and good farming practices, both at county and state levels. His sons now carry on with his same traditions.

After rearing our four children and working the family farm in Eastern Oregon, John and I were looking forward to enjoying our golden years together. At the age of fifty-three, John was diagnosed with Alzheimer's disease and our plans were disrupted. This abrupt change in our lives, sixteen years ago, resulted in John's retirement and my suddenly becoming a caregiver.

The farm and his family were John's life so it is good that he has been able to still live on the farm and be a neighbor to two of his sons. He probably doesn't understand what that means, in the normal way, but hopefully some recognition is still there. Optimistically, I feel that John still knows this deep in his heart.

Not knowing and learning how to go about my daily task of caring for a child-like adult has been an unusual adventure. It has become a daily challenge to figure out how to avoid problems before they happen or at least how to quickly solve problems when they do arise. I have learned to take one day and each challenge at a time.

People were continually telling me that I should share my solutions to our problems because of what I have learned from my everyday experiences. I never considered doing this until I read that my local community college was offering a night class called: "Writing Your Life Story." I decided that perhaps I was meant to write about my daily problems and how I learned to handle them. Sharing our story seemed logical because of the help it might offer to other caregivers and because John and I are both middle-aged so I still have the stamina to try to figure out how to solve caregiving problems as they develop. If John and I were both in our eighties and still healthy, it would be all I could do to just take care of our daily requirements and anything extra would be more than I could handle.

We do wear many hats in life and my styles have evolved and changed over the years. I feel blessed that we are able to be together and the sickness and health part of our marriage vows can still be lived. I try to be grateful for what we still have.

I have told our story of the past sixteen years in the order in which the digression of the disease developed and I have tried to update John's progression backwards as they have happened during the two years of writing this book.

Statistics have been added as I felt they would be necessary to help another caregiver understand the full extent of Alzheimer's disease and make them more knowledgeable in general if this should be the only book they read. I certainly could have used help as I learned to become a caregiver. If I can now share my experiences and help someone else it would be very gratifying.

My sense of humor is really what has gotten me through this period of life. I hope you all have one. You will need it to help keep you both laughing.

PROLOGUE:
LIVING BEYOND THE JOURNEY

John was a farmer from Eastern Oregon when I married him fifty years ago. He loved making things grow and found joy in simplest things in nature, the quiet of early mornings, the whisper of wind across the fields, and the beauty of the Oregon Trail ranch where he was born.

Together, we raised four children to value hard work, believing it was the best gift we could give them for their future. Though farm life demanded long days, we never missed an athletic event or school activity. We worked harder on other days, but family always came first. Ours was a simple, grounded life filled with purpose and joy. As the children grew and started families of their own, they blessed us with nine wonderful grandchildren. Two of our sons even returned to the farm, joining us in tilling the soil and tending the cattle. Life was good, full, and deeply rooted in the land we loved.

Then, in 1983, everything began to change. John was only fifty-three when discontent and anger crept into his personality. By the following year, he grew passive, withdrawn, and uninterested in daily life. His short-term memory began to fail. It was difficult to convince him and even harder to convince doctors that something was wrong. But an MRI revealed extensive brain shrinkage, and the diagnosis of early-onset Alzheimer's disease came swiftly. It felt like a death sentence to me. Thankfully, John never fully understood it. From that moment, I resolved to take life one day at a time, just as the saying goes.

As the disease progressed, John seemed to travel backward through life, first as a young man, then a teenager, then a child, and finally like an eighteen-month-old baby. In the spring of 2002, pneumonia ended his journey at home, at the age of sixty-nine. Although his death certificate listed pneumonia as the immediate cause, I knew in my heart and from sixteen years of watching him fade that it was Alzheimer's disease that truly ended John's life. He had no cough, no fever, and in the final two days, he lay quietly in bed. There was no sign of pneumonia attacking his chest. I had to insist that Alzheimer's be added to his death certificate so future generations would know the truth of what he endured. I share this not only to honor John's legacy, but also to remind other families that they have every right to insist on the accurate recognition of Alzheimer's as the cause of death. My greatest fear had always been that he would face many long, bedridden years, but that was not the path before us. Perhaps I learned through this that borrowing trouble from tomorrow only robs us of today.

My goal was always to keep John mobile and active. Daily walks helped him nap peacefully and rest through the night. I am convinced this routine kept him healthier for longer, improving circulation and keeping him engaged.

People often said once an Alzheimer's patient entered a wheelchair, they never got out again. By God's grace, we avoided that fate until the very end.

Of course, caregiving brought challenges that tested me daily. Incontinence became one of the greatest burdens, both physically and financially, but over time I learned how to manage it. Wandering was another constant struggle. John lost all sense of fear and reason, and I had to protect him as one would a small child. Sometimes he would hold my hand and let me guide him, at other times, I had to gently 'herd' him. I gave him simple responsibilities, like holding my purse or coat, to help keep him seated in public places. Covering a doorknob with a towel or jacket made him forget it was there, preventing him from slipping outside unnoticed. On warm days, I let him walk outside barefoot or in socks, the gravel slowed him down, and he quickly learned to stay on the cement and deck.

Small adjustments became lifesavers. He could still feed himself, so I cut food into small bites and gave him a medium-sized spoon. I cooled his soup with crackers to make it easier to eat, and I never gave him caffeine, which only kept him awake at night. These may seem like little things, but each solution brought us one more day of peace together.

As the sixteen years unfolded, I learned not to take anything for granted. I solved problems one at a time, always with love and determination. Eventually, friends encouraged me to share my story. I never imagined myself writing a diary, let alone a book, but I realized they were right. When John was diagnosed, I had searched for practical, one-on-one guidance and found very little. So, I wrote Living with John: Caring for a Loved One with Alzheimer's Disease in hopes of offering comfort and help to others walking this same difficult road.

The response has humbled me deeply. Readers have told me they passed the book through twenty members of their family, reading it as if it were a novel. Their interest and compassion touched me more than I can say.

I hope my story reminds you that you are not alone. Every caregiver faces heartbreak, exhaustion, and fear, but also moments of tenderness, strength, and even joy. John's journey taught me that love can outlast disease, that patience can grow deeper than despair, and that courage often appears in the quietest acts of daily care.

If my experiences help even one family cope a little better, then John's legacy lives on, not just here on the farm, but in every heart that continues to fight Alzheimer's with love.

DESCRIPTION

The American Medical Association describes Alzheimer's disease as a neurological disease with loss of short-term memory and reasoning power. Alzheimer's has been called "the death of the mind." Alzheimer's causes the death of the brain cells that allow us to make necessary connections for the thought process. As a result, memories become unglued or fragmented. The person forgets what they used to know and can no longer retain new information. Our healthy brain mass from ages twenty to seventy loses only ten percent of that mass.

Usually a patient's life span, following the beginning of the disease, will range from three to twenty years. I have even read of patient's living with Alzheimer's for up to thirty years.

Alzheimer's, sometimes referred to as AD, is named after the German doctor, Dr. Alois Alzheimer. In 1906, Dr. Alzheimer noticed changes in the brain tissue of a middle-aged woman who had died of an unusual mental illness. He found abnormal clumps, now called senile plaques, and tangled bundles of fibers. Today these are considered hallmarks of Alzheimer's Disease.

Different specialists will use a various number of stages such as three, five, or even seven stages to explain different symptoms and the progression of the disease. The naming of stages is changing now as doctors are finding vast differences in how and when individual patients go through each of these stages. This was also true in John's case. The medical profession's explanation of the stages did give us a guideline to go by. This has also helped me, as a caregiver, to know what the future symptoms might be, allowing insight as to what I could expect next.

The people, who work with Alzheimer's patients, will most often identify the disease in three phases: mild, moderate, and severe. Keeping in mind that the divisions are approximate, they can overlap and sometimes vary from patient to patient. These three phases can be viewed as follows:

MILD SYMPTOMS:
Stage one -- may last 2-4 yrs. or longer:
- Confusion or memory loss
- Disorientation; being lost in familiar surroundings
- Problems with routine tasks
- Changes in personality and judgment

MODERATE SYMPTOMS:
Stage two -- may last 2-10 yrs.:
- Difficulty with activities of daily living, such as feeding and bathing
- Anxiety, suspiciousness, agitation

- Sleep disturbances
- Wandering, pacing

SEVERE SYMPTOMS:
Stage three -- may last 1-3 yrs. or longer:
- Loss of speech
- Loss of appetite; weight loss
- Loss of bladder and bowel control
- Total dependence on caregiver

The Alzheimer's patient rarely remembers a last thought, whereas a healthy person often recalls later that what they could not remember or what was just on the tip of their tongue. A well-known example of forgetting is losing or misplacing the car keys. Such forgetting is normal for all of us, the dementia patient however does not know what the keys are for when he does find them.

An aged healthy person is usually able to follow written and oral instructions and can even write notes to themselves to remind them of things that they might be prone to forget later. A patient with Alzheimer's gradually becomes unable to follow written or spoken instructions. For example, he eventually is unable to read labels placed on his sock drawer for the purpose of helping him recognize where the socks are located. John in the very early stages of the disease lost this ability to comprehend.

When John was first diagnosed, the doctor said he might possibly have Pick's disease, a different type of dementia, and only time would tell. A patient with Pick's disease deteriorates very quickly leaving no short term or long term memory. An Alzheimer's patient however is believed to retain long term memory, while losing short memory. Years later, I saw a man with Pick's disease. He was in his early forties and in a nursing home. He behaved as a person possessed. He was in the dining room playing what looked like musical chairs by himself with no music playing. He could no longer recognize his wife or small children soon after the diagnosis. The experience made me realize how truly lucky we are. I like the thought of John remembering his childhood on the farm with his parents and four sisters, or having early memories of our four children and myself.

John and I traveled frequently the first few years, when he was still able to enjoy seeing the areas of America that earlier he could only dream about while driving a tractor all day. Months later, John would refer to something that had happened on one of our trips. I did not understand how this was possible with a short-term memory problem. When I asked our nurse, she said it was no longer short-term memory that he was experiencing, his recollection was now stored in his long-term memory bank. I was pleased to hear that our brains had this capability. As John walks around all day, I like to think that he is still remembering our trips to Texas and New Mexico, or possibly a funny childhood situation.

I have read that John will eventually think of me as his mother. When I think of this idea, I guess I really do not mind it at all. Gladys, John's mother, was a wonderful human being and was much beloved by her son.

SYMPTOMS

Unlike a newborn baby awaiting a long and healthy life, a person with Alzheimer's disease experiences the reverse process. Alzheimer's works backwards through the process of life, with the end resembling the beginnings of life. The patient is left with the mental and physical abilities of a newborn.

It is important that all of us be aware of warning signs that could be precursors of Alzheimer's disease. It is now recommended that if your loved one is displaying any of the dementia symptoms listed below they should be started on the prescription drug Aricept or the herbal Gingko. These are safe preventions while the diagnosis is being decided upon and may help to slow the symptoms in the early to moderate stages. This drug or information was not available in time for John so please take advantage of all the new knowledge. The problem will only get worse, don't try to ignore it. If I can't help in any other way I would like to impress on families the urgency for early diagnosis.

The Alzheimer's Disease and Related Disorders Association, Inc. published what I believe to be a very helpful list of the 10 Warning Signs of Alzheimer's Disease. I am listing them here for your reference.

- RECENT MEMORY LOSS AFFECTS JOB PERFORMANCE
  Everyone forgets things and then recalls them later. An Alzheimer's patient forgets often, never recalls and reportedly asks the same question, forgetting the earlier answer.

- DIFFICULTY PERFORMING FAMILIAR TASKS
  People with Alzheimer's disease could prepare a meal, forget to serve it and forget that they even made it.

- PROBLEMS WITH LANGUAGE
  A person with Alzheimer's may forget simple words or use inappropriate words, making speech incomprehensible.

- DISORIENTATION OF TIME AND PLACE
  People with Alzheimer's can become lost on their own street and forget how they got there or how to get home.

- POOR OR WEAKER JUDGMENT
  Even a normal person might be distracted and fail to watch a child. A person with Alzheimer's disease could entirely forget the child under their care and leave the house.

- PROBLEMS WITH ABSTRACT THINKING
  Anybody can have trouble balancing a checkbook; a person with Alzheimer's could forget completely what the numbers are and what is to be done with them.

- MISPLACING THINGS
  A person with Alzheimer's disease may put things in inappropriate places—an iron in the freezer or a wristwatch in the sugar bowl—and not be able to retrieve them.

- CHANGES IN MOOD OR BEHAVIOR
  Everyone has occasional moods, but people with Alzheimer's can have rapid mood swings from calm, to tears, to anger- within a few minutes.

- PERSONALITY CHANGES
  A person with Alzheimer's may change drastically and inappropriately, becoming irritable, suspicious or fearful.

- LOSS OF INITIATIVE
  People with Alzheimer's may become passive and reluctant to be involved in activities.

John and I lived with the early signs of Alzheimer's for a couple of years before his disease became evident. Convincing John that he needed to seek medical help was my first big hurdle. Denial is a very large part of the first stage for both the patient and those around them.

At the beginning, before we knew there was a problem, John's personality went through a variety of changes. For instance, he fired a hired hand; Larry had worked for us since he was a boy in high school. John came home and told me all about it saying, "I have taken all the lip from him that I am going to." This was very unlike John. He had always been very satisfied with Larry and had never fired anyone in his thirty-five years of farming. I felt bad about John's letting the boy go but now Larry is a man and again on the farm working part time for our son, Scott. Since all those around us understand our situation, I know that I could call on any of our two son's hired men for help in an emergency and that is a comforting thought.

John became very self-centered. If something took his fancy he did it. Another day, John announced to me that he was going to do as he wanted and it did not matter what anyone else thought. He proceeded to do just that.

No matter which television show I chose it seemed to be the wrong one. If I cooked chicken, he was hungry for hamburger. I finally just waited to start the meal when John arrived home to avoid arguments. During this stage, he began salting everything at the table before he even tasted it. I had always seasoned food amply in the kitchen and this was something unusual for John to be doing. He didn't want to listen to me that salt can be bad for your body because we were getting older and there is always a worry about high blood pressure and heart disease. I just got a salt substitute and put it in the shaker. By letting him have all the salt he wanted, it seemed to satisfy either his changing taste buds or John's urge to defy me. This phase seemed to slip his mind after a while as so many others have over the years as he goes from one symptom to another of Alzheimer's disease.

John even began to eat food off my plate with no explanation. He seemed to believe it was his right. I have read that eating other people's food in the early stages is a symptom in some patients. John slowly was becoming a textbook example.

Deception becomes important in an Alzheimer patient's lives. They do not understand what is happening to them and will try to cover their confusion in such a way that it may go undetected. John became a master of turning situations around so that the problem became my fault. He argued constantly about everything to the point where I began to question my own sanity. By passing on the blame for all that was happening in his life that he didn't understand, I think John was trying to hold on to his own identity as a powerful and strong-willed person that he felt was seldom wrong. He was now making mistakes that a small child could do right and it depressed him. John's personality was quickly slipping away from him, and he did not understand why. Neither did I. I'm sure, at this point, with all the arguing our children wondered what we were doing still living in the same house. It was not a happy time for either of us.

I questioned John about these changes in his behavior. He had no answers, with sadness and confusion he just replied, "I don't know." At that time, I felt a doctor would have sent John for psychological help. Somehow I felt that was not the solution, as John did not act as a mental patient would. This stage of the Alzheimer's disease lasted for about one year. John seemed not to be concerned with problems of daily living during this period.

On one occasion, I noticed a small round, callused hole on the bottom of his foot and found the source inside John's cowboy boot. The new heels had a nail going up through the heel and into the inside but John continued to wear the boots daily that way, just putting up with the annoyance by ignoring it.

I had never been given any reason in all of our married years to suspect John of fooling around but out of desperation to solve our problems, I asked John if he had found another woman. I knew infidelity would be extremely hard for him to live with mentally, as he was always a very moral and straight-laced individual. John quickly assured me that this was not the problem and he had no idea what the real problem was. Actually, I believe infidelity would have been a simpler solution and something that we could have solved one way or another.

The second year, his personality seemed to go into neutral and John seemed to turn inward. During this stage of the disease he acted as if he was on tranquilizers. Life was so calm and peaceful after the previous year that I went around just keeping to myself for fear of our lives changing for the worse. Our lives did, but not the way I had expected.

Later I felt guilty for not figuring out John's dilemma and getting him to a doctor sooner. Dementia never occurred to me at this time, as I believed Alzheimer's disease was for older people. John and I weren't old. At that time the general public knew very little about the disease since the patient's physical well being could often be very deceiving and John's certainly was in great condition.

During the third year, different subtle clues began to appear. It was just a matter of picking up on them. This was the time many of John's lifelong friends wondered what they had done to alienate him. He was distant and not the usual fun loving extrovert he had always been. John even loved to go to weddings, just to visit with his friends at the reception. He now wandered around as if in a daze.

John's short-term memory had begun to deteriorate. He could not look up a telephone number in the book and remember it long enough to dial. This was one of the first symptoms of the disease that John asked me to help him solve; even then I didn't realize we had a problem starting in our lives.

Money was also a new problem, as amounts seemed to be completely confusing for John. He started leaving two dollars for a tip, whether he had a soda pop or a full meal. I began giving him our Visa card to pay the restaurant bill. John could still sign his name until the late middle stages of Alzheimer's. I suppose our name is one of the early things we learn and that is why John's signature was so ingrained in his memory. He seemed to want to be in charge of this situation and that little piece of plastic solved our problem for about a year. This maybe helped him to feel valued and competent in some way.

We were living with the various symptoms, but because of the lack of public knowledge, I knew very little about the disease and nothing about the possibility of early onset.

Years later, Alzheimer's disease is now getting closer to a breakthrough and because of public and government research money; it is often in the news. I read the other day of a test for the disease. I, unfortunately, heard of this test too late to help us but I try to inform others who are concerned about their loved ones. Have the patient draw the face of a clock on a piece of paper and then ask them to put on a time, such as twenty minutes to three. If it looks fine, they may just be having short-term memory loss typical of most of us as we age. If it looks like apiece of modern art with the numbers out of sequence, there is the possibility of Alzheimer's disease and they need further testing. Judging the passage of time is one of the first losses to occur. In order to know how much time has passed, you have to be able to remember what you did in the immediate past.

DIAGNOSIS

About the third year into the disease, I pleaded with John to see a doctor but he continued to insist there was no problem. I could see John was getting worse. The problems were growing and piling up fast.

As an Area Director of the Pendleton Grain Growers, a local farmer's co-op, John was requested to serve as master of ceremonies for Hermiston's annual meeting. He had done this often over the years and John always handled it like a professional. I tried to explain to the organizer that John was going through some changes we did not understand and I felt John would not be able to speak that year. The caller argued, insisting that the speech would be written out and John only had to read it. Against my better judgment I gave up and agreed. John felt there would be no problem. The night came and as John stood up at the head table to speak, he suddenly had no idea what to do. The chairman had to take over for John at that point. On our way home in the car, he looked over at me and said, "You're right, Nellie, I think you should get me a doctor's appointment." I felt this has been a rude awakening but maybe necessary to clarify in John's mind there really was a problem.

In order to see the neurologist in Walla Walla, Washington, John had to be referred by a local doctor. I took John to see a new doctor who had recently replaced our retired, original doctor. After a thorough examination and physical, the doctor said, "This man is as normal as I am." I became very alarmed and told him we needed help as I lived with John daily and recognized all the symptoms of Alzheimer's disease. The doctor acted as if I did not know what I was talking about and I became concerned. I did a very female thing. I cried and I begged the doctor to get us an appointment for an evaluation. He told his nurse to call the neurologist. I am sure he just wanted to get me out of there. We never went back to him.

We traveled the seventy-five miles to see the specialist in Walla Walla. After a lengthy discussion with John and I about our lives, the specialist felt we had no problem. John was still able to carry on a normal conversation. By this time I was desperate. Knowing we could not return home without a diagnosis of some kind, I went into my concerned wife role and insisted he perform the testing anyway. The doctor told me to wait outside and he would do it. After about thirty minutes, the doctor called me back in and with surprise in his voice said, "He has a very bad short-term memory loss!" I asked, "What are we going to do next?"

The clinic put John through a battery of tests lasting all day, beginning with a check for low levels of vitamin B-12, one of several causes of dementia in the human body. The B-12 test was normal so they proceeded further with an EKG and an EEG then completed the testing with a MRI. The possibility that another disorder may be causing the symptoms must always be eliminated. The symptoms associated with Alzheimer's disease can mimic stroke, minor head injury, effects from high fever, poor nutrition and certain drug overdoses.

Medical researchers are now saying that a microscopic injury to the brain can cause trauma and may be linked to the development of Alzheimer's disease many years after the injury. This study will lead to renewed commitment to educate the public about behavior that will reduce the risk of head injury such as wearing seatbelts while traveling in an automobile or wearing helmets while riding a bicycle or motorcycle. It has also been proven that soccer players are more prone to the disease later in live than other types of sports player because of the headhits involved. Any blow to the head that has caused temporary unconsciousness is very suspect. John has never suffered from any of these. He did have a bad spell as a teenager due to sunstroke while stacking long hay. John worked out for long periods in the eastern Oregon sun mid-summer and became sick and he said, "The next thing I knew, I woke up and the priest was giving me the last rites." If this high fever and unconsciousness had any affect we will probably never know as no one has ever asked any questions concerning his childhood. The more I read it seems that will soon be changing for newly diagnosed patients. They have to find a common thread and who knows that history better than the victim and their family?

John and I returned home about six that night. The doctor phoned shortly afterwards. He said the good news was John did not have a brain tumor, but there was bad news: his brain was badly shrunken. I asked what that meant and the doctor told me to return to his office and we would discuss it another day. I told him to just tell me over the phone. He said it meant that John had Alzheimer's. There was no indecision in his voice.

John and I saw the doctor a few weeks later to discuss Alzheimer's disease. I asked him not to explain details of the course of the disease to John. The doctor disagreed but honored my request. I had read enough since the diagnosis to decide there was no reason for John to hear of the dreary and bleak future ahead for the both of us.

ACCEPTANCE

It is often said that writing your own life story is cleansing to the soul. While this may be true for some writers, I am not finding it particularly uplifting. To describe what has happened in our lives is interesting, yet depressing at the same time. I will try to explain the feeling to see if this helps in any way. There is something to be said about taking each day at a time. Thinking back, it seems even more overwhelming probably because I am reliving those years and experiences all at one time instead of a few each day.

I cried for three days after the diagnosis. This gave me an understanding of the three days of mourning experienced by those who have had to live through the death of a loved one. I needed that time to say goodbye. John, as he had been, was gone for all of us. I made up my mind after those first three days to accept what time we had left together and to make it as livable as possible for both of us.

Between crying bouts and moments of feeling sorry for the both of us, I would feel better and call another relative or friend to inform them of our diagnosis. Each time I put the three words together, "John has Alzheimer's," I would fall apart and ask that person to call others. This was the beginning of my new support system.

Life may not be perfect, but three days after John's diagnosis of Alzheimer's I thought of several disasters that I felt would have been much worse. A brain tumor, because of the pain involved; a car wreck, ending as a quadriplegic; or a massive stroke, causing him to live in a vegetative state. After that realization, I accepted and prepared to live with the hand we had been dealt.

Recently our friend, Betty sent me a saying on a card entitled *ATTITUDE* by anonymous. The part of it I liked best that I will share is the following: "The longer I live, the more I realize the impact of attitude on life. The remarkable thing is we have a choice every day regarding the attitude we will embrace for that day. We cannot change the inevitable. I am convinced that life is 10% what happens to me and 90% of how I react to it. And so it is with you…We are in charge of our attitudes."

Being an eternal optimist helped me to come to this decision those many years ago and probably helped to save my own peace of mind. Alzheimer's Disease has been referred to as "The Long Good-bye" or "The Living Death." I refuse to view it that way. I feel John is still with me in body and spirit even if his mind has slowed over the years. Everyone ages; his aging has just gone a little faster.

Acceptance of John's disease was still hard no matter how optimistic I tried to be. We had four grown children who were taking the news very hard. Our three sons also had spouses and nine children who would also have to live with this new happening in all our lives. As farmers, we had spent a lot of quality time with the four children. Our lifestyle had allowed this. John had worked daily with his three sons on the ranch. The loss of the guidance their father had always given them was going to leave a large hole in their hearts and lives. Our daughter, Valerie had been in Europe after getting her doctorate there and she decided to return home to be closer to her father. So all our lives were disrupted but I really appreciated the family support.

About the third night after John had been diagnosed, as we were lying together in bed, he mentioned the disease for the first time. John asked, "Well Nellie, the doctor says I have Alzheimer's what are we going to do about it?" I said, "We're going to live with it and take each day at a time, I will take care of you, so don't worry about it." Relieved he said, "Okay." John then peacefully rolled over and immediately went to sleep, never to mention it again. I rolled over and quietly cried knowing at that moment how alone I was.

CAREGIVING

When I first learned that John had Alzheimer's, I was completely ignorant as to what the disease would mean to both our lives. I felt faced with a future of nothingness. I am now trying to fill that void for the many people who are in my situation, and for all of those who will follow. If I could have read about another caregiver's first-hand experiences twelve years ago at John's Alzheimer's disease diagnosis, my life since would have been much simpler. Knowing then what I do now would have eased my worst fears.

I would like to give support to those caregivers who are caring for their loved ones at home or providing care and love in an alternative living situation, such as nursing or foster homes. You should consider joining any support groups that are furnished through your loved one's organization or if you are caring for the patient at home join through your town or church. If there is none, consider starting an association. Knowing you aren't alone is of tremendous help mentally.

After I had read all I could find in the local library, a total of two books, I was very discouraged, mainly because

I was looking for some common sense. I checked the same library ten years later, and they still have the same two books. One of which is a child's book, *When Grandpa Doesn't Know Me Anymore*.

Several books that our son, Mark, purchased at an Alzheimer's Association meeting in Portland such as *The 36-Hour Day* helped but I found little that was really practical to help us with everyday living. If I were to read these books now at this stage of John's illness, I would probably utilize the advice in an entirely different way. With that in mind, I recently reread *The 36-Hour Day* and can see why I felt I received no help from it twelve years ago. It is a great reference book for each problem as it arises but reading it completely before really understanding the problems referred to in the case histories did not assist me at the time.

Resources were written primarily about how to diagnose the disease and then how to select the right nursing home. Two of the books I read were written primarily for nursing home caregivers and included how to handle family visitors diplomatically. This was interesting but not an immediate concern of mine. Daily living help or maybe just a few words from someone in the same situation were what I needed so I wouldn't feel so alone. That has been one of my main concerns and goals with writing this book.

Caregiving is difficult when the person you are caring for doesn't recognize his need for care or appreciate the caregiver's efforts. I'm sure paid professionals appreciate family members telling them, "thank you" on occasion because their loved one no longer can.

Everyone has a horror story to tell. When I read a story that included a caregiver's wondering, "Who would have ever thought that she would eat the marbles in the bottom of the fish bowl?" I thought then that I had read enough. There were some things I just didn't need to worry about until they happened in some form or another. Since then so many of those strange incidents have happened. I believe that every patient will act out in his or her own different and individual way.

One of the first questions that people will ask me is if John is mean to me, since that is what they often hear concerning Alzheimer's disease. I told someone the other day when they asked me this, "No, but I'm sure he still remembers that he wouldn't get away with throwing me against a wall twice!" Actually, I read somewhere that only about one in ten patients get a violent personality change. The use of unnecessary aggressiveness is often when loved ones can no longer control the patient and decide to put their spouse or parent into a nursing home where tranquilizers are incorporated into the daily regime.

People think I am courageous and strong, because I have decided to keep my husband at home, rather than taking him to a nursing home. For us, in my mind, alternative care is not yet a decision that needs to be made in our case. When the time comes that I can no longer take care of John, then I will do what I feel is right for both of us. In the meantime, I do what needs to be done now, as I grow further into my role as a caregiver. Family and friends should not be concerned about my health. We have four children who are making sure they don't lose their mother, as they no longer have their father as he was.

As long as there is a glint or even a hint of a human being still lurking behind John's eyes or as long as I can still get a chuckle out of him I will hang in there. To explain to others that this way of life is really the best way for me is difficult. If John were not home, I would be making the fifteen-mile trip into town to the nursing home daily. I know I would be sitting in a depressed state with him or walking him around the facility, wishing neither one of us was there.

The stress of changing an Alzheimer patient's natural environment takes a huge toll on them, both emotionally and physically. Familiar places and routine experiences are essential for maximum functioning. Alzheimer's patients often have trouble just adjusting to an overnight motel stay.

Not putting John into a nursing home does not mean that I am an exceptional wife. This is simply the way I feel life should be for us. Home is where John and I both belong, quietly going about our daily lives: he in his dream world, me in the role of wife, homemaker, and now caregiver.

My only nursing experience was as a volunteer hospital aide at the Multnomah County Hospital in Portland, fifty years ago, when I was a Girl Scout. Cleaning empty rooms, feeding people who were blind and elderly or powdering surgical gloves made me realize there was more to the medical profession than caring for happy new mothers eager to see their babies. Now, as a caregiver, I feel fortunate I at least had that training and experience. Often in the early stages of John's disease, I felt a strong need for any help to fortify me for the problems that I had read would lie ahead for both John and myself. I was also glad that I had First Aid training and can perform CPR or the Heimlich maneuver if either should ever become necessary in John's later stages.

The following list of skills is listed in the National Alzheimer's Association booklet to help the caregiver by informing us of the tasks that we are likely to face:

- Providing adequate supervision
- Ensuring patient's medical well-being
- Providing for patient's financial security
- Assisting with household chores
- Assisting with personal care
- Providing support or companionship

Many of these points have been touched upon in this story of living with John each day and throughout the years. This is my personal version of how I have managed. It is my hope that some of the solutions will be of help to the reader.

RESEARCH

I knew enough about Alzheimer's to realize it was a slow demise backward through life, with no known cure. After John's diagnosis, 'cure' was the word I seized upon and decided to get more information.

The association states that studies of Alzheimer's disease can be divided into three broad, overlapping categories. The first is research on causes, the second is diagnosis, and third is treatment, which includes caregiving.

The morning after John's diagnosis, I called the National Alzheimer Association's number 1-800-621-0379 and was told they would send me their pamphlets. I asked about any research being developed in the Pacific Northwest and they mentioned a large hospital in Seattle, Washington.

I called the Seattle hospital and spoke with the doctor doing the research. After I explained our problem, he told me the drug they were testing was not performing as they had hoped. He told me not to come over the mountain for this drug and said that it was not doing as well as he had thought it would. I was almost relieved we didn't have to drive over the Mt. Rainier passes during the winter months in our little car. The doctor was referring to Cognex; the first drug put on the market because of patient and family insistence. It seemed to help some patients in the early stages, but it also can cause liver damage, which meant frequent blood tests.

There is now another drug available, Aricept, which helps the patient much the same as Cognex without the liver side effect. I currently have John in the Aricept program even is it is mainly for the early to moderate stages and his has gone beyond that. Just in case it can still help him we are going to try, as I feel there is a lot they are not certain of with Alzheimer's. My understanding is that Aricept is a short-term answer as it is most effective during the first six months of usage and like most drugs helps only certain patients. Other medicines will be on the market in the near future. Ibuprofen is being recommended to take a one tablet a day dosage to possibly prevent inflammation in the brain area but it can also give liver damage over a period of time in some people. Patients or caregivers should ask their doctors about any new drugs that are available that they think might help a particular client.

The same month as John's diagnosis, we were able to get into a research program at Good Samaritan Hospital in Portland. The first drug John tested just had numbers for a name because it was so new. They thoroughly tested John's word knowledge by holding up different articles. He did fine with glasses, pens, scissors and so on but had trouble with forceps each time. John would be given words to remember and repeat a few minutes later. Even I had trouble doing that! They were always amazed at John's ability to copy drawn figures of intertwined squares and horizontal forms. It is very hard for the patients to work puzzles, screw nuts onto bolts, or do several things in a row, after hearing the series of instructions. These tests were given each visit as a way of measuring the disease's progression.

We made the four hundred mile round trip every week for six months, then every other week for six months, every three weeks, and then once a month. You can see I was determined to do all I could to find a possible solution to our problem. I don't enjoy driving at all and mainly like to travel when it is to new and different places. Thankfully, the Columbia Gorge in Oregon is one of the most scenic routes in the United States because we saw it in every season of its glory.

We were going to Portland once every three months and were on the fourth drug of a research program, hoping for the one that would help John in any way possible. We went for a new supply of pills and to explain any unusual symptoms that John might be experiencing. The drug company was to provide a lifetime supply of the drug he had been taking, since we had proved it helped John during the research stage. We have received word recently that the manufacturer is no longer going to produce the drug and John has been removed from the program. It did not slow the progression of the disease but seemed to give him a very manageable and happy personality.

The research coordinator was surprised that John had been as stable as he had been for the last three years. We do not know if this is due to the drug, genetics, or the one-on-one care I give him daily. Maybe it's his feeling of freedom and continuity derived from living in the country with lots of space and a great view overlooking his farm and past life, who knows?

John's symptom of Alzheimer's occurred before age 65, so his disease is called early onset and is often considered genetic. The first thing I read after his diagnosis was the younger you get it, the harder it hits, and the faster it progresses. That bit of information really hit me all right, the hardest of all my reference work, as I had expected John to live to be into his hundreds. Both sides of his family are very long lived, so genetically he should have lived to be a very old man like his great-grandfather, who at the turn of the century, died at the age of ninety-four.

But fortunately the early demise has not been true in our case and I encourage all people diagnosed with Alzheimer's to get into a drug research program as soon as possible. Someday the medical profession will have answers. We were told about nine years ago that a major breakthrough would probably happen in ten years. This may be too late to help John, but hopefully it will help the predicted millions.

RECOGNITION

Even in the early stages when John was at the research center and was being asked a lot of questions; he was never sure how many children we had. I do feel however, that he recognizes his family even today. I will never forget my sad feeling when they asked him if it was his wife sitting beside him and he said," No." Then they asked him if I was Nellie and he said, "Yes." I like to think the problem was with the word, wife. He had lost the meaning of that particular word but still knew me as a person and that fact was what was important.

It has always seemed unusual to me that the first thing most people will ask when seeing us after a period of time is, "Will John still know me?" I assure them that they always meant a lot to him. I actually am wondering where they have been all the past years. He would have enjoyed a ride to town with them or they could have just stopped by for a visit to say, "Hi, how are you two doing today?" Little things might have helped him hold the memory of them. It also makes me sad that I do not have the nerve to explain how I really feel about the situation, but I ask myself, "What good would it do?" Then I recall how important it was to me that he knew who I was, so maybe it is a natural reaction for all of us to want to know the answer to that question.

If I sound cynical, I am sorry, but at times it does get to me. I try hard too not let it and I tell everyone that it does not. On my fifty-fifth birthday, which was a long eleven years ago now, I bought myself a tee shirt that had a cow lying on her back with its four feet in the air. Underneath it read, "Really, I'm fine!" I got it, because when I saw the shirt, I realized that was what I had been saying for the past year. Actually, I was also teats up but I felt down deep that no one wanted to hear it. They just wanted to know if John would recognize them. If, as a caregiver, you sometimes feel depressed or alone, you should. People with a "normal" life style do, so why shouldn't we? Alzheimer's disease can be as frightening for the caregiver as it is for the person who has the disease. It is probably more so for the caregiver as we know more clearly what the future holds for both of us.

As the years pass by, I am beginning to realize that this could still go on for a long time and John would not want me to devote myself so thoroughly just to his care. I am getting better about taking a few hours or even days occasionally for myself. We have a friend who is doing the self-sacrifice routine and it has opened my eyes to what I had been doing for so many years. I am now trying to adjust my lifestyle and hopefully she will also soon be able to let go a little at a time.

As a caregiver, we certainly are not alone. The Oregon

Alzheimer's Association states that statistically 76,000 of the four million people afflicted with Alzheimer's disease are Oregonians and Oregon has the fastest growing elderly population of any state west of the Mississippi. The number of Oregonians older than 85 is growing six times faster than any population group.

Alzheimer's can continue from three to thirty years or more and medical help costs the nation one hundred billion dollars a year. The federal research budget is three hundred eleven million dollars a year.

We were lucky to have our will and estate planning in place before John's diagnosis. That is something that is easy to let slide by each year by assuming we will live forever. We also applied, after the diagnosis, for social security disability and we did have to put in for it twice. The bulletins state that this is the usual way it is handled and to just not give up. Our government is slowly making us all have to become as tenacious as a pit bull in order to have our rights as a taxpayer fulfilled. We had paid into the system for years as farmers and I knew that it was also my future support as John's wife and partner. Nursing home care can strip a family's investments fast and so can an early-enforced retirement.

We immediately went to our lawyer to get our power of attorney transferred into each other's names. I did it that way so that John wouldn't worry about the procedure and wonder why it had suddenly become necessary.

Everyone will eventually be touched by this disease, so research is working hard to be able to diagnose it in the early stages. They are trying to find the solution or at least slow or shorten the length of time involved in the progression of the disease. Almost every week the newspapers or television mention some new breakthrough that will hopefully lead to the final answer. They, of course, first have to find the cause before they can find the cure.

Just this October of 1999 the news headlines were the findings by U.S. scientists believing that they had isolated the elusive enzyme responsible for the build up of plaques in the brain, a hallmark of Alzheimer's disease. The discovery could lead to new treatments for the disease as well as ways to determine who may be at risk for developing Alzheimer's. They also said the development of the drug would be years away but it is a major breakthrough towards a cure.

MEMORIES

John has never cared to visit the rest of the world but seeing the United States was something he had always wanted to do after he retired. There was no choice, ready or not, now we were retired. I knew we needed to build memories for both of us and we did not have a lot of time in which to do it.

Within a few months of John's diagnosis, we began our tour bus trip adventures. I liked the idea of the travel decisions being made for us by a guide, because I was daily making all other decisions. In addition, riding all day, just watching the world go by really pleased John.

My mom was in her late seventies and early eighties during this time and had never had a chance to travel. She had always kept the books at my folks' automotive part supply business in Portland but now my two brothers and their wives run the business, so she was able to come with us. Having mom along was fun. She seemed to really enjoy herself and mom helped me to keep an eye on John at the same time. Later when she could no longer travel with us, my younger brother, Dick joined us for a couple trips and we saw new country together.

John's behavior was manageable enough when we first started our traveling experiences. During the beginning trips to Arizona and the Canyonlands, we did not tell any one of his disease. As the Alzheimer's progressed, I told the tour leaders and the bus driver because John was becoming confused about some things, such as which bus was ours. Usually we got along fine. John had always been the social one of the two of us so he could be happy just sitting on a bench watching people pass by in front of him.

In the beginning during long periods on the bus, John would sit and read a western novel. Then on one of the trips, I noticed that he had the same page open all of the time. It was then that I learned he could no longer comprehend what he was reading. A patient with the disease explained in a television interview that when she read she could no longer remember the part that she had just read. Since she didn't know what had happened, none of it made sense any longer so she gave up all reading. This was just what John finally did.

I started checking out audiocassettes from the local library and John would happily listen to the books he could no longer read. We still listen to tapes on our short trips to town and our longer trips to Portland. John will even laugh in the right places and sometimes the wrong places but the main thing is he really seems to enjoy the stories.

John always liked being with a group and people accepted him willingly. Later on, when he tried to join in conversations, some of his comments did not make any sense. I remember a man once said his daughter had been accepted into a certain college. John asked, "How do you know that?" This was his often-used addition to a conversation, and was probably due to the fact that there was so much he himself no longer understood. At those times, I would explain our situation. By then people knew us and did not consider him an oddity but us as just a couple with an unfortunate problem.

As we were only in our fifties, we were usually the youngest of the tour groups. I think that we may have brought out some parenting instincts in the others. They were mature enough to be very understanding and often had been around Alzheimer's disease. They knew it could hit any of them or their loved ones at any given time.

It was younger people who had a tough time understanding the disease. John could no longer comprehend the menu at a restaurant. I would place his order for something I knew he had always liked and for food that was easy to eat. John's favorites had always been fried shrimp or chicken-fried steak. The waitress was used to a man ordering so she would ask him what we would like and I would answer for both of us. The looks I would receive varied from "bossy to bitch." When I did bother to explain, the term Alzheimer's disease usually meant nothing to them during those early years.

I became frustrated enough that I designed two pins to wear. One said "caregiver" and the other said "care receiver" with an interesting logo for people with strokes, mental disabilities, or any other dilemma. The idea for the pins was to let the public know that one of the people had an illness and to refer questions to the caregiver and to treat the care receiver with the respect that they deserved. I went as far as to get a patent but never found the right place to develop the idea. Several companies just returned all the information and said there was no need for it at that time. If they only knew how helpful it would have been to a lot of caregivers for identification purposes.

Thankfully, the disease is better understood now. People coming forward such as former President Ronald Reagan at age 83 in 1994 has helped the rest of us, not just with research dollars but also with compassion and understanding. He aptly described it as, "Beginning the journey that will lead me into the sunset of my life."

There was a news story about a man who knew President Reagan who said, "I don't go to see him because I want to remember him like he was." The often forgotten fact is that it's not about one's own comfort zone but about the afflicted person and his needs. Nancy Reagan says she is living "step by step," which is so true in most anyone's time of adversity. What better time to show your friendship and love to both people involved, the caregiver and the patient. Remember that they both are traveling down an often very long and lonely road.

INCONTINENCE

Unexpectedly, our travels came to an abrupt halt. We had flown with a tour group to the Great Lakes area to see the Ameri-Flora flower show. I believed this would be a fun trip for all of us. My mom had graduated in 1931 from Washington State College in Landscape Architecture, so flowers have always been one of her loves. It was early spring and Holland, Michigan was ablaze with tulips.

It was a great trip, but coming back John got off the plane with wet pants. From then on, incontinence became a part of our daily lives. John not only had bladder problems, but also soon developed bowel difficulties. All of the charts that I have read on the different stages of Alzheimer's disease put incontinence in the last or fetal stage. John had started this in the late first stage. I believe this is one of the reasons the medical profession has given up on the typical stages. Each patient is as different as children are in their intelligence, development, and achievements.

I try to remember to put John on the toilet after naps, meals, car trips and during the night. Sometimes it works, but often it does not. When we were away from home, I would send him into the men's restroom and he would return immediately without having time to have used the facilities. At unoccupied rest stops, I would go into the restroom with him to get the job done. It isn't always easy to locate that ideal situation. The Lloyd Center shopping mall in Portland has a special family restroom just for such situations but it's one of the few that I have seen. Maybe future demands will change and solve this problem as the handicapped are being brought to the forefront and their needs considered more each year.

In the early stage, I kept a night light on in the bathroom to encourage John to get up in the night when necessary and of course to help him see better when he did. We often had a wet bed and I finally decided to try a variety of absorbent pads. There is a selection in sizes and prices depending on where you buy them and the quantity purchased. The larger the box, the less expensive they are. The latest in adult briefs has a gelling property that absorbs more urine than fiber-filled materials and is less bulky.

So we would not have to worry anymore about wet outer clothes while in public, I bought rubber pants. I also bought several night undergarments to help keep the bed dry. I have collected a large assortment of pads to put on the bed, such as used shower curtains, old cut-up plastic sheets and crib-size absorbent pads. They are all inexpensive and effective.

Luckily, John has never gotten any body rashes. I keep diaper rash ointment in case it should ever become necessary. Whenever he is wet, I change him as soon as possible. I also use a baby wipe every time he gets up from the toilet because there can be a smear left that I can't see. If his skin becomes irritated at all, John doesn't want me near him the next time and then I have to chase him all around the bathroom to clean him up and I have learned to keep the door closed or he is long gone.

If I had my way, *POOP IS MY ENEMY* would have been the subtitle to this book because of my experiences with several situations. I won't go into any of them here as I know you have either, as caregivers, had or will have, your own times in poop hell so I knew that you would understand but that the publisher wouldn't and I was right. Just know that you have my sympathy in this area.

When John is first seated, it is easier to remove the used pads by cutting the side tabs with scissors rather than trying to tear the plastic apart. I then place the soiled diaper into the sink because it is an easy place to clean and use anti-septic on later. I have learned with time that there is a lot of waste when using incontinence absorbency control. The patient often wets in just a small area. While the pad is still in the sink, I cut out the dry parts and use them as inner pads on the next dry replacement just as you would use a sanitary napkin. This has been quite successful and I wish I had thought of it years earlier. I probably save every third pad by doing this.

I then carry the soiled pad parts to a lidded outdoor hamper. I can later burn the pads with my daily garbage collection. I know this is an advantage because we live in the country.

I prefer small babywipes for bowel cleanup. The adult sizes seem a waste, as they are too large, and because sometimes the pads are awkward to use. Using thin wash cloths in anti-bacterial soapy water is a good finish to the skin and helps to prevent rashes. I furnish disposable gloves for substitute caregivers but use disinfectant soap on my own hands for cleanup. If John is really a mess, I clean him up in the shower. This is the easiest solution to a bad situation.

When rediapering a man, the most important thing is to make sure that his penis is in a down position or he might as well not be wearing a pad.

John sleeps in two absorbent pads, a washable cloth outer diaper and a plastic one over all. He sleeps on a cloth pad over a plastic one for comfort and protection.

We have a king-size waterbed and that saves the mattress. It is recessed with wooden railings, so he cannot fall out onto the floor. John fell out of bed once when he spent a night at a nursing home. He was found sitting on the floor in the middle of the night and he had to be examined for physical injury and luckily there was none. I have known several women that have broken their hips that way and then the attendants put the railing up on the side of their bed. It always seems like closing the barn door after the horse has left to me and seems like care is what you are paying for. Our nice warm bed is not foolproof and I do have to change the entire bed sometimes in the middle of the night, after wiping the mattress with a disinfectant. When this happens and our sleep has been disturbed, we just sleep a little later in the morning.

Once, after I complimented a nursing home on their lack of odors, they informed me they use a product made to destroy pet odors. I purchased a spray bottle of it and have used it on carpets, blankets, etc. Sometimes I spot wash so I don't have to wash the entire article. I use white vinegar in the wash machine, and in spite of trials of other products, I think that vinegar is the most economical and effective method of removing odors from the soiled garments. If I have an all white load, bleach does a great job. Washing the soiled nightclothes and bedding each morning prevents a smell throughout the house.

Several years ago, John got out of bed on three different occasions and wet down the leather-padded chair in his clothes closet. When I read that Alzheimer patients sometimes mistake other objects for the toilet, I changed that chair, after the second accident, to a bright, colored, plastic one. The first two times I ranted and raved, and was ashamed of my lack of patience. When it happened a third time, I handed him a sudsy wash cloth, and more or less forced him to clean up the chair as I would a naughty child. I felt guilty afterwards, but he never mistook anything else for the toilet again. I must have gotten my point across. I have wondered though if he was pushing me to see how far he could go by seeing what I would actually put up with from him. I often feel there is a lot more understanding behind his haunted eyes than one might think.

The main thing I have learned is to expect the unexpected and to take nothing for granted.

DRIVING

Whether or not to let John continue to drive or not, was our next big hurdle after the incontinence. We own a farm and knew that we would definitely be liable, if by any chance, he had an accident and was at fault if someone was hurt or even killed. We had worked very hard, at low wages, to keep the farm in the family and we did not want to lose it through a lawsuit, let alone cause anyone injury. As a family, we felt that after the diagnosis, we would be at fault because we knew of his problem. I asked a lawyer about this and he said at this time there was no law that would force an Alzheimer's patient to quit driving but thought that someday there would be. Statistically it is known that people seventy years old have four times more accidents than the average person but we were learning that there are several reasons why some drivers should never again get behind the wheel.

We had tried to drive through San Francisco and it was easier to let John drive at that time then to let him try to read a map that he could no longer understand. This happened in the very early stage before I realized our problem was that extreme. John drove to Portland several times on our weekly doctor visits and did not seem to mind the traffic or have any trouble. After a few months, I noticed he was questioning where to turn and did not seem to want to believe the traffic signs, let alone me. I would just have to insist he turn at the right exits.

As the disease progressed, I began to worry about him finding his way home while driving alone. We live a considerable distance from the three local towns in which we do business. Even a familiar environment changes day by day. Being lost seems to be a common problem with patients even in the early stages, so I decided to explain to him all of our concerns.

I cut up his driver's license in front of him for emphasis. I explained that he could drive all over the farm but he was not to ever go out onto the highway. I then had to purchase a new identification card from the motor vehicle's department because I wanted a good picture I.D. on his person in case he was ever lost or in an accident. John no longer carries any identification as I was always washing it when it was in his pocket because I always forgot to check them. I decided his safe return bracelet would have to be enough. He also has identification name tags ironed onto his clothes whenever he is away from home and me.

Only once did he drive off the ranch and that was almost a year later. I was in the hospital because of stomach problems and we had planned a trip for the next day. I had told him earlier that we would get his hair cut before we left. He just showed up where I get my hair cut and said he had an appointment. He didn't but the beautician cut his hair anyway. He then proudly came and showed it off to me. You can be sure that my mouth fell open.

I mentioned earlier that this disease works backwards through life. As teenagers we learn to drive and boys especially love to do just that. John was an excellent driver and because he had grown up on the farm he was driving all of the equipment at a very early age. Our sons noticed that he now drove very fast and listened to loud rock and roll music, just as a teenager would, when he drove the many roads on the farm. This was no problem until he pulled up to close to a tractor in the shop lot and took the side mirror off his pickup. At that point he seemed to decide, with our son, Kent's suggestion, that he should not drive anymore. We removed all the keys from the ignition switches and I did all driving after that and John never again got behind the wheel. It was sad for him to lose that part of his independence. He accepted it better than a lot of men would have and I was proud of him. To this day, he will sit in the car in the garage hoping it will take him on a new adventure.

We went through several jumpstarts and a new battery before I finally got the automatic door lock on his door disconnected as it was drawing just enough electricity to be a problem. Earlier I had removed all of the light bulbs but the battery would still drain down and the car couldn't start. This always happened after John had left the door open overnight and we couldn't understand why the battery would still be dead the next morning. The mechanic thought there was nothing left to use up the electricity but we eventually found out that there still was and fixed it. That was one problem I was very glad to get solved.

John may not drive anymore but he definitely still likes to sit up front. We have tried to put him into the back seat of a club cab pickup a couple of times and ended up with the feeling he would be there the rest of his life. We would have to almost bodily remove him. He now gets to sit up front!

Sometimes it is hard to convince John that the trip is over and that it is time to get out of the car. I usually have to take his pants cuff and pull out the right leg and then the left so that he gets the idea the trip is over and we're home. If he continues to stay there in spite of this, he eventually gets out of the car on his own. He has now stopped ever getting out until I take his hand after I pull his legs out and help him. If it is necessary that he get out immediately and he strongly refuses to help me at all, I will lie down on the front seat and push him out the door with my feet. This is not very lady-like but sometimes I have to do what I know will work but I try not to have to do this in public.

Nothing makes John happier than riding in the car. I sometimes wish that I liked to drive more. We could go and go and go until we arrived back in the past, where we were the happiest.

HYGIENE

Habits of personal hygiene are lost early in Alzheimer's disease. Remember Alzheimer's makes its movement backwards in development and what little boy wants to wash behind his ears?

John had always brushed his teeth three times a day and they were pearly white. They slowly turned yellow after he refused to brush them and he would not allow me to go near his mouth. As his disease progressed, I learned if I put an object in each of his hands; I could brush his teeth. I usually do it at bedtime and in the morning after his shower while he is still sitting on the toilet. I use an anti-plaque solution with fluoride toothpaste, hoping that will help. The brush I use is an extra wide one to cover more area in a shorter time. He seems to enjoy the process after I get it started. I took him to a geriatric dentist in Portland to have his teeth x-rayed. I wanted to make sure he didn't have infection going into his system from abscessed teeth. They did fill several of his front teeth at the root area but were afraid to drill inside of his mouth. They were emphatic about daily brushing and I have tried to do that and they do look better than they did. John was born on this farm and the wells all have extra hard water so luckily he has very few fillings in his mouth.

John had always been insistent about everyone shaving, even on hunting or white water rapid trips. Because of this, I felt it would be a blow to his vanity to let his beard grow. When he would no longer shave himself or let me do it, I finally gave up and just let his beard do its own thing. By that time he did not care anymore and actually it is quite becoming. We had tried to go to a barber, for both a beard trim and a haircut, but John would become restless if they took too long. It was not long before I had to sit on his lap to hold him on the chair. Rather than experience the mounting embarrassment that accompanied this process, I decided to keep John at home and do my best to trim his hair and beard. I had always cut his and our three sons hair while growing up, as they are all curly headed, so mistakes cover themselves over. I now use a comb and scissors, again, while he is sitting on the toilet. Usually John is the most cooperative at night when he is very sleepy. Rubbing his head or massaging his neck also seems to help put him into a receptive mood.

This is also where I cut John's fingernails and toenails. I have learned to put an object into each of his hands in order to prevent him from pushing me away while accomplishing any of the aforementioned procedures.

John dresses and undresses himself while sitting on the toilet. He likes to zip up his pants, fasten the button and buckle his belt while he is still sitting down. I then have to undo these before he can stand back up but it is entertaining for John and good practice. I try to get him to continue to do as much as possible for himself. My belief is that the more often John can do something, the longer he will hold onto those learned memories. If I get him started, John still knows how to button his shirt, pull on his socks and zip up his pants but now these are also fading from his memory.

Sometimes I have to tickle John's calf so that he will remember to lift his leg when I put on his pants. He can still tie his shoes, which never ceases to amaze me. I realize this simple skill is one we all learned early in our lives and we continue to use every day throughout our lives. I am sure this has helped his long-term memory bank. Not knowing when this skill will leave, I now buy him shoes with Velcro closures to speed up the dressing process.

I am always careful to tuck John's tee shirt into his pants or he will finger the edge of it while he walks around. If I don't tuck the shirt in, John will eventually manage to tear a hole in it and then he really has a good time. He looks as if he is trying out for the lead part in Streetcar Named Desire.

During the first stage, John would get out of bed early each morning and take a shower. He always said, "Taking a bath is like sitting in your own dirt." Since he was a farmer, that was probably true and I never knew him to get into a bathtub. At this stage, he could still shower himself. I was pleased about this until I got up and watched him one morning. All he was doing was holding his hands out, catching the water and then opening his hands, letting the water fall to the floor of the shower without ever getting any on the rest of his body. I have no idea how long that had been happening.

Now, when it is time to shower, I help him by heating up the water in the shower stall and warming up the room. Then, I turn off the water. Before he enters the shower, I put both the shampoo and conditioner, at the same time, on his dry hair and beard while he is still sitting on the toilet. At this time, I give him a nice head massage. He acts like a dog that cannot scratch his own itch.

I scrub his fingernails with a brush dipped in a liquid type of soap. I make this soap mixture by taking various scraps of bar soap, placing them in water and leaving them there until they are liquid. I hate to waste things and this is a good way to use the small pieces of soap. We get a lot of them because John spends more time washing the bar of soap then he does himself. I then hand him a bar of soap, being watchful that he does not try to take a bite out of the soap. He can chew it up before I can get it back out of his mouth. This gags me but does not seem to bother John.

Next, I head him towards the open doorway of the shower. I have read that some Alzheimer's patients will not go into the shower stall because they seem to think it does not have a bottom and they will fall. At one time, I had to chase John around the bathroom with the toilet plunger in order to get him through the shower door. This was our bathing process for quite some time. It seemed to be a game to him and soon became a daily ritual with him running around chuckling and me quietly chasing after him trying to herd my bull into the right gate. I always have that visual as I can't push or pull him but have to guide him from the rear any time that I am trying to get him to go where I need him to be. As cattle ranchers we spent a lot of time trying to get animals through openings and at certain times I find myself using the same technique with John. Now, he goes into the shower stall quite willingly and seems to thoroughly enjoy the experience of the warm water flowing over him.

It is very important to turn down the water heater to 120 degrees in order to protect the patient against burning. This way, with the hot water faucet turned on with a small amount of cold, the water is the perfect temperature and I don't have to worry if John changes it. I hold onto the spray nozzle while I am standing outside the shower door. John washes his bottom and genitals by himself. He never cares about washing anything else, so I soap the rest of him down and rinse him. He rubs his hair well while I hold the sprayer over his head to remove the shampoo. This is probably just because it annoys him when I get water in his face.

I am always thankful that he can still help me as much as he does. If I give him a towel and leave the room, he will usually step out of the stall on his own. Otherwise, I step in behind him and put my hand on his back and he steps right out willing to be dried. He will use the towel on what he still considers his most important parts and then I will dry the rest of him. While he is again sitting on the toilet, I dry his hair, put lanolin on it and brush it while it is still damp.

Because of a bad back, I usually get down on my knees in order to help with socks, pants and shoes. I often lift his leg across my one bent knee for support. I go monthly to the chiropractor to get a vertebra alignment as I have three herniated disks in my lower back and that doesn't help my situation.

It is becoming harder to get John to sit on the toilet, despite the fact that I bought a nice padded seat for it. After I help him pull down his pants and pads, I push down on his head and gently push in on his stomach. Sometimes, he sits right down and at other times I think we could make a lot of money on one of the video contest shows. I am on his back trying to get him to sit. He is either pushing down hard just above his knees or holding on to the edge of the bathtub, laughing. Lately, I have again been putting something in each hand, which helps. I am still winning but he is very strong and determined. Because of the aggravation, I find that I do not take him to the bathroom as often as I used to, so maybe he is winning.

WANDERING

John has always been in excellent physical condition. This is still very much the case. He has the body of a high school track star at the age of 66. He is living proof that walking is a great exercise because he does that all day long. He takes our stairs two steps at a time while I am dragging myself up by holding onto the banister. Our son, Scott, says that I should follow Dad around all day for exercise. That's easy for him to say!

The experts call the pacing that John does "wandering." His behavior fits their description perfectly and he has now done it for many years. One doctor said it is his way of replacing his job. As a farmer, he was always on the run going here and there all day moving irrigation hand lines, digging out the flood channels, running down newborn calves and general farm work from dawn to dusk and that is what he is still doing. Some psychologists believe wanderers are running away from an intolerable present reality. I prefer the job version, as John was always happy and proud to be farming. He had worked long and hard to be able to leave the land to the third generation of Madisons that his father and mother had homesteaded.

Gaylord and Gladys had, slowly over the years, bought out the adjoining homestead farms. They and their children did without in order to keep this farm in the family and not lose it to draught, taxes or low crop and animal prices.

I have learned over the years that I can get John to remain sitting in a chair if I give him my purse or coat to hold onto while he is sitting there. It is as if he feels he then has a purpose to stay seated and perhaps he is doing something for me, his caregiver.

If I put a towel or coat over the doorknob on the door, he will usually walk past it and not remember that it is the way to the outside. I have also read that a mirror placed on the door works well. The patient evidently sees someone coming towards them and turns to go back the other direction to avoid them. This is because in the later stages, they do not recognize themselves, while looking into a mirror. Several years ago while visiting a friend in the nursing home, John walked past a mirror, looked into it and as I watched him I realized he was looking at nothing familiar. His eyes were totally blank.

If I take him to a caregiver respite center, everyone is sitting quietly in chairs along the wall all around the room. Not John, he is busy walking all over the place and is always attempting to get out of the front door. It is hard to find a care center that is secured well enough for wanderers. The first place I left John they assured me it would not be a problem. When I called to see how he and they were doing, they asked me to return for him as two attendants were standing by the door to keep him from going out into the busy street. I have only left him at gated facilities since that time. They are few and far between because you can't lock everyone else out or others in so it means an entirely separate unit. We don't live in an area with enough population to warrant it evidently.

Many patients both in and out of nursing homes become especially restless towards evening. The medical term for this is "sundowning." It is not known if this happens because Alzheimer's patients seem to be tired and therefore harder to manage after the long day or maybe they become frightened when it gets darker outside, as there is a lack of sensory stimulation. The routine noises are a major source of security; so many patients sleep well only during the day and in chairs close to the nurse's stations.

John will walk all day but he does increase his pace after supper and before bedtime as the evening progresses. He sleeps all night and this makes me think that all the daytime activity helps to tire him. I encourage a nap after lunch, as I know John must be tired and in need of a couple hours of rest so that he can get up and go again. It is up to the caregiver to learn the patient's fatigue level, I make sure John rests enough to restore his energies.

When I asked John's nurse at the research center, four years ago, what would happen next, I was told he would start staying awake all night. Thankfully, that time has not yet arrived. I know how important my rest is to me and probably more so for John because of his constant activity. I have learned to lie down for a quiet time myself, during his nap, to help refuel my own energies.

I used to let John walk on the farm. I would always put an orange vest with reflective stripes on him before he left home to help me be able to see him from our house. John always stayed on a road, but would never turn around and come back. Only once did I see him turn around towards our house and that was because the irrigation circular sprinkler was crossing his traffic pattern. John watched it for a long time then finally turned and came back up our hill.

One time after looking all over the ranch for John, I found him out on our back desert road on the far end of the acreage. I asked him if he wasn't tired and he said, "Yes I am." I asked him then why didn't he just turn around and come back home, as he could see our house on the hill. I will never forget the look on his face when he answered, "I don't know." Those three words were the same ones that he had used years before when I had first asked him what his problem was.

After nine years as a caregiver, I had a heart attack. Because I did not have any of the typical risks for heart trouble, the doctor immediately assumed the high stress of my caregiver role was the primary reason but I did not believe that was the case. A clean angiogram later proved that my heart attack was probably due to a blood clot. I was told I had been very smart to take two aspirins, when I felt the first symptoms and that it had probably saved my life. The medical news on television last month announced that research has suggested that a person with heart attack symptoms should take one aspirin immediately. It was reported that if this were done, one thousand lives a year would be saved. I was told years ago, that if my symptoms ever returned, I am to put two aspirins in my mouth and chew them and then swallow. Then I am to put a third one under my tongue with the nitroglycerin tablet that I carry but have never needed to use. I have told this to everyone that will listen, as I am telling all of you readers now. I also take daily a coated aspirin to keep my blood thin as the doctor says that some blood just magnetizes together and probably that is what happened in my case. Women fear breast cancer and we are much more likely to die of heart attacks.

Just in case the doctors were right about my stress, I decided that the most straining part of my caregiving life, at that point, was locating John on the farm after his daily hikes. I tried to buy a locating device to help me find him but there was no such thing on the market at that time. I have tried to compensate by going with him on his walks but walking has never been high on my list of fun things to do. Thinking of any reason to not do it is easy but I am trying to get a more positive attitude and take more walks with him. I know it would be good for both of us. My lack of interest comes from walking a mile to and from school daily, rain or shine, up hill both ways, as my grandkids say, when they quote me. The bus picked up the neighbor kids one house further and if I knew then what I know now, I would have walked over there and got on the bus.

How to keep John from wandering away from our yard suddenly presented me with my newest problem to be solved. I finally realized that he would not walk away from the house if I just took off his shoes. He soon learned that the gravel was painful in just stocking feet. He seems to have forgotten his leaving home days and now I can use leather bottomed slippers so he does not wear out all his socks and they help to keep his feet warmer. It also cuts down on the leaves and debris coming into the house on the bottoms of his socks. Luckily, the house we built sixteen years ago has many doors and rooms that flow from one to the other. There is a wooden deck, which has a wonderful view and gives him a good walking area. Apartment dwellers must find it very hard to care for a wanderer and I appreciate daily how lucky we are.

To live with damaged thinking and judgment is to live at risk. Cars are a big problem for wanderers. Even on our early bus trips, I had to hold on to his arm at intersections to keep him from stepping off the curb into the line of traffic. In the early stages, I asked the doctor if John would actually do just that. He answered, "Yes, he will because, like a child, he won't know enough to look to the right or left for cars." Now I guide him in the right direction. He was always a gentleman and took my arm, so he is used to walking with me in that way and is very cooperative. John seems to have no concept of danger and this really worries me. There have been a couple times that we have found him on the highway walking on the yellow centerline as if he was Dorothy seeking OZ.

The night before taking a trip with John, I can count on having a nightmare in which I lose him and it is always in a very crowded area. Then I spend a restless night looking for him. At times it leaves me so tired that I question making the trip. This is the only time I have such nightmares. Obviously, losing John is a very big concern and must be on my subconscious.

Knowing how much John likes to travel, I always take him to town with me. He sits in the car with his seat belt on and the door locked. I can keep an eye on him from inside the store and he can watch all the people come and go. This is possible because I have a handicap-parking permit from the Department of Motor Vehicles. This worked fine for a long time. Then one day, I came out with our groceries to find the car door unlocked and open and John pushing an empty grocery cart all around in the busy parking lot. When I called his name, he turned and looked at me and pushed his cart as fast as he could in the opposite direction just like a disobedient two-year-old.

I then had a new problem to solve. So John would forget it was there, I decided to cover the seat-belt release button so he couldn't see it to push and then leave the car. A paper towel roll and a toilet paper roll were both too small, but a map tube fit perfectly. I cut it about four inches long and slipped it over the short end of the seat belt closure. When the belt is in place, I just pull the tube up and over the release button. Now I am confident that John will always be in the car when I return. So far he has been and that has been several years ago now.

John also does what is called "shadowing." It could drive me crazy if I let it, but I make sure that I do not as I realize to him I am his security. Anywhere I go in the house, John is right behind me. He will even get up from the table, quit eating, and follow me into the utility room or wherever I am going. I just visit with him and consider it is company for us both.

He still enjoys watching our grandkids play the various sports each season such as football, volleyball, basketball, baseball and tennis. It seems that as long as someone else is moving, John does not have to move constantly himself. We don't go to the away games anymore because I realized about four years ago, that John seemed to be afraid of the open spaces under some of the bleacher seats. Our home gym is solid seating and we always sit in the same area just inside the door. He is used to us doing the same thing each game so that consistency may help to make it feel familiar to him.

John used to watch the players as they ran down the court and his head would move back and forth. Last year I noticed that he was spending most of his time "people watching" those around him. It is hard to get him to look at anything far away, even through a car side window, as he always looks straight ahead.

Sometimes being smarter than John has been a challenge. I try not to expect anything, as I never know what he will do next. All we can do is wait and see what the future will bring for both of us. The fact that John is still as mobile as he is such a blessing that I try not to let it become a problem in our lives.

SAFE RETURN

National Alzheimer's Association statistics show that 59% of those with Alzheimer's disease or other dementia's will become lost and that 46% of those not found within 24 hours of the time they were last seen -- may die. During the winter months hypothermia presents a particular risk, as the temperature drops and it becomes dark earlier.

One of the best gifts we ever received was the gift of peace of mind because of a birthday present given to John. Our daughter-in-law, Shannon, signed him up for the "The Safe Return" program through the National Alzheimer's Association. It is a system that assigns each participant their own identification number through computers to all the applicable police stations.

John received an identification bracelet with his own I.D. number and the words "Memory Impaired - to help John, call" 1-800-572-1122. On the front it says "Alzheimer's Association Safe Return." We also received a number of nametags with John's I.D. number and the 800-telephone number imprinted into them. I use these for laundry tags on all the clothing that goes into his respite care suitcase. John could wander away from anywhere, not just from our home or car.

I heard the other day about a man with an Alzheimer's affected wife and he was so concerned for her that he also wore a safe-return bracelet. He felt that way if anything should happen to him the medics would know to also check on her. I thought that it was a clever idea and a possibility of something I should consider.

I actually did lose John once for a half-hour at the Lloyd Center, a large shopping mall in Portland. Without my noticing, he went in a different direction and when he wants to he can really move right along. Often he would walk ahead of me and end up standing by a group of people, staring at them and listening to them talk. By the time I caught up with him, they would be wondering, "Who is this man?" I would explain our problem, and we would walk on down the mall.

This time, however, he was nowhere in sight. When I couldn't see him, I immediately returned back to the immense parking garage because in this middle stage of his disease, our car seemed to be the most important thing in John's life. He was like a homing pigeon, as far as the car was concerned. I usually found it easiest to just let him find our car in the parking lot and I would follow him to where I had left it earlier. This time there was no sign of John and I was beginning to panic. He could have gone out any exit door and then I would have really lost him, out into a very large city.

My mom was with us, so I left her inside the mall to keep watching for John. When I could not find him anywhere, I returned back to the area where she was supposed to be and she was gone. This was my first and only time that I have had to request the help of a security guard. He immediately radioed to the rest of the guards to be on the lookout for both of them. It was not long before I spotted John walking one flight below me in the mall. Luckily, he was not inside one of the stores, or worse yet, outside the mall. We returned to the area where my mother was going to wait. After a while she returned and I asked where she had gone, to which she replied, "The lady's room, up two flights." Such things are necessary, but it sure was bad timing. We notified security and left for the car and safety.

This experience made me think again about our Safe Return program and I realized the information I had sent to the National Alzheimer's years earlier was now very outdated. The first thing I did on returning home was to update all changes. As John aged, his hair had become grayer and he was now wearing a full beard. He no longer used glasses, as they were always either lost or filthy. They had been a very weak prescription for distance and not that important for his everyday vision. These changes could make quite a difference while trying to locate someone in a crowd. If it should ever become necessary to find John, it is important to have recent information for the police. I also sent them a recent photograph showing the new changes in his appearance.

Losing John was as an eye opener for me, and made me realize just how quickly and easily a person can be lost. My only security was the fact that he was wearing his Safe Return bracelet. I highly recommend one for everyone in case you have a relative who might decide to leave you at the dog races. Seriously, the terrible fact is that it is estimated between one hundred and two hundred thousand patients are abandoned in emergency rooms of hospitals each year. This is a sad testimonial to the compassion of the American people.

PHYSICAL AGING

Although Alzheimer's disease is a neurological problem, some of John's first symptoms were physical, as well as mental. Months before he was diagnosed, he lost about one-third of his hair. On his paternal side, there is very thick, tight, curly hair. John's hair suddenly became thin and wavy. It is still that way. The doctor said that hair loss was not a symptom of dementia. This, I thought, was the reason he ordered an M.R.I. as he suspected a brain tumor. I have learned recently that there is no connection with hair loss due to either disease so John's hair loss is still a mystery to me.

Before his diagnosis, John also became sensitive to temperature, especially the cold. When we were in the car, he would want the heater on high. I was starting menopause and was already too warm. This was a complete reversal for both of us. We had become Jack Sprat and his wife. I think that he is cold because his blood pressure is normally low and the research medicine he is on can cause lowered blood pressure. John used to take nine pills a day. He is now down to three because his blood pressure is only 100 over 60. I assume he is colder than the rest of us because of this. I put a set of wool socks and long underwear on him to wear during the day and to sleep in during the winter months. He wears flannel shirts or sweatshirts daily except during the summer. These help to keep him warm and are important to his comfort.

John's doctor warned me years ago that it would be up to me to figure out by his symptoms if he was having any signs of an illness. He said John wouldn't even be able to let me know if he was having a heart attack. So far we have been very lucky with his health, as he has not acquired any of the typical old age diseases. Having Alzheimer's Disease won't exempt him from any of the others.

John had never had skin trouble until the last time I left him in a care center for a few days. He is usually happy there for about three days. After a longer period, it seems he feels I have left him forever. Since John's last stay of one week, he has had psoriasis, which is a stress related skin disorder. I am told he will have the patches of dry skin, off and on, for the rest of his life. John is usually calm and happy, so I hope I can keep the psoriasis under control.

It seems the last few years are aging John faster than normal, maybe three years for each one he lives. I have read nothing about this being typical but it makes sense as the body's functions begin to shut down and the disease progresses in the brain. I wish there was some way to collect observations and speculations from patients and caregivers throughout the United States. The statistics could then be put into a computer and analyzed for common occurrences among all patients. It might even help to find a common cause and cure.

In his late fifties, John's toenails became very thick and yellow, as a much older person's would. Is this common? I have no idea. Another unsolved mystery; someone must know the answer. Maybe I am just supposed to accept all the strange happenings and not wonder about them, but knowledge is comforting. I just try to keep his toenails and his fingernails trimmed to prevent him from scratching himself.

John's gait sometimes varies throughout the day. He does not always pick up his feet well anymore when he walks, another reason he wears slippers with soles in order to save what is left of his socks. Last year, he would have left the house in slippers, but he has only tried to leave a couple of times this year. I am sure that he does not remember that he can still leave home if he so desires. He often goes outside and looks down the driveway and stands and stands until I come and call him to come back in the house. I don't know if he is dreaming of going somewhere or if he has just come to the end of the cement and can't turn around on his own. As the disease progresses, John's need to be near his caregiver seems to increase, as it probably was in his childhood and maybe this keeps him home.

I have a kiddy gate at the top of the stairway to keep John upstairs. This helps me know where he is, as he will not open the gate. If I leave the gate open, he usually goes downstairs and stands by the bed and throws back the bedspread even after I have just gotten him up in the morning.

John waits for me to help him into bed. I think this started a few years ago because when he would get into bed his head would be lying up on the headboard and he would be sitting on his pillow. He would have to get back out of bed and I would stand between him and the head of the bed and push him down and over onto the right area. Perhaps he's decided he cannot please me, so he just waits for me to help him.

He also stays in bed until I help pull him out of it. It seems I have become his alarm clock. I warn our children that if they don't check on us occasionally they will find two bodies dead together because if I have a heart attack he will stay right there in bed beside me. It is like all families, as each one probably thinks that the other is taking care of the situation.

They would do anything for us, we just have to ask and that is the hard part, isn't it?

This thirteenth year John has become more sedentary. Before, I would have to sit on him to hold him in a chair just so he could get a few minutes rest. Now he will walk around and then sometimes sit on his own. This is good because he gets more rest this way but I am sure it probably also means he has declined and is physically more tired.

I am afraid he has slipped a little farther into the deep pit of his disease and his future is progressing backwards through life. He is fast approaching the fetal stage. When

John first returns home from a care center, he will sit more, maybe because everyone there was sitting. He may be encouraged to do the same, as then he is easier to watch.

NURSING HOMES

One of the consequences of Alzheimer's disease is the need for full time care, often in an assisted living facility or nursing home. If you are lucky, you planned for this eventuality and purchased long term insurance while you were still healthy. John was so healthy at 53 it never entered our minds.

Many people do not realize that Medicare and regular health insurance do not cover long term care. About 40% of all nursing home expenses in this country are paid for privately and about one-half of the expenses are paid by Medicaid, the government program designed to subsidize patients who cannot afford long-term care.

Nursing homes have been a big help in my life, but they have also presented me with new problems to solve. During John's first visit to the local Alzheimer's care facility, I learned that he was getting very little sleep. The day crew assumed he was sleeping all night and the night caregiver thought he was up because he had been napping in the daytime. Actually, he was doing neither. Unless someone puts him to bed and goes through his regular nighttime ritual, he is wandering around. That is his job now and he does it very well.

I learned I had to be very specific about John's particular habits. The turnover in nursing care help seems to be almost weekly. Even the caregivers that do stay are three nights on then four nights off with three changes of staff daily. This makes for a variation of caregivers in a week's time. When I leave specific instructions with the first person, it seems to go no further, hence the taped instructions by the bedside for staff changes seems to be helping. I feel I need a second one as to his eating habits for the lunchroom. On his last visit, they gave him a napkin and a hot drink and I had specifically requested neither. I know they have a lot to look after so I just need to help in any way that I can without becoming a nuisance.

A nursing home caregiver, about 22 years old, approached me once and mentioned how much she had enjoyed taking care of John. She stated concern, however, that he would not let her give him a shower. I asked her if he would let anyone else help him shower? She answered, "Yes, he did let the older woman help him." I immediately knew the problem was that she looked like a Barbie doll and no way was she going to see him nude if he could help it. It is interesting how the mind of an Alzheimer's person does maintain certain images. In his own way he was trying to retain his pride.

The first time John went to a home in Pendleton I was assured that they could handle a wanderer. My granddaughter and I settled him in the downstairs area that was specifically for Alzheimer's patients. We were getting in my car to go to Ashland, when whom did I see heading out through the parking lot towards town? My peace of mind was very short lived. John had gone out a basement door into the walking area, up a ramp to the upstairs, and out the front door. The nurse, who had assured me that she would always be at that door, was "on a break." It was a wake up call to us all. I called the next day to reassure myself that they were being more observant by then, which they were.

Another time he did not sleep because he was sharing a room with a new patient who got up every few minutes, turned on the light, and left the room to walk around. That was John's cue, and he was reported to have shadowed behind the patient all night long. He evidently felt his new roommate was his new caregiver, therefore his security in his world of insecurity. John looked ten years older when I returned just days later. I have tried to get him a private room since that incident and have asked the caretakers to close his door, with the lights out, when they put him to bed. He is still very social and thinks that if there is something happening, he should be in on it.

One time I came home to a husband who looked as if he had lost at least ten pounds. His arms were much thinner and even our grandson asked," What's wrong with grandpa?" The nursing home personnel informed me this time that he had just quit eating for no apparent reason, just as he had at home several times. Assuming they had expertise in the area of Alzheimer's, I had not informed them about using a straw in a cup of liquid to start him swallowing again. When I do get him to start eating again, it means hand feeding him three meals a day for a while. This becomes very time consuming as he eats each bite so slowly and will not take a second bite until he has swallowed the first. People who say you should chew each bite fifty times would love him! I already do love him, or I would have chucked it in long ago.

After my marriage I became a gulper. My husband and four kids were ready for dessert before I had finished my main meal. Consequently, I do not have a lot of patience when it comes down to hand feeding and try to keep John able to do this for himself. Meals must be very time consuming for nursing homes. I often hear of family members going in to feed their loved ones at least one meal a day just to be sure that they are getting proper nutrition.

The last nursing home at which I left John for a few days told me on the second day, when I called them and wanted to see how they were getting along with him, that there was a problem. When I asked with concern what it was, she said, "He is pacing very fast while looking in all the rooms and out the door windows." I told them to remember he was a wanderer and in much better shape than the elderly that they were used to, so he did walk fast and he was still trying to find me, his caregiver. I didn't worry about it any longer because if I did, it seems that my respite would be a waste of time. I knew the facility could keep him clean, healthy and out of harms way because that's what they do. Nursing home employees are a very dedicated group of people and they all have my admiration, as I don't think I could handle it for very long.

It seems that I have done a lot of fussing about the care John receives while in nursing homes but really I do appreciate their availability. I am mentioning different experiences we have had, so that anyone who has a loved one that they can no longer care for at home, will look for certain symptoms when they visit. They can call it to the attention of the attendant, then check the next visit to make sure that the situation has been improved and is being taken care of properly.

A recent research project on nursing home care showed that dementia patients using a rocking chair on the average of an hour and a half a day improved sociability and helped to prevent depression by elevating their mood. It also helped the patient improve their balance. If this works there it should also be of help in the private home situation.

If you are observant, it is still possible to give one-on-one care to your relative, even in a professional home. No one at the facility can be expected to know the patient's own particular needs and desires as well as the family do. We have to remember that our loved one is one out of a number of patients to them.

I have always felt if each of us would care for one elderly or ill person, things would balance out and everyone would have someone. All you have to do is let your friend or relative know you are there for them, remember them on their special days, and then make other days important. They are happy with little things and it does not take a lot to be a bright spot in their lonely day. A visit to your local nursing home is not always a pleasant experience but one must consider the mental well being of the people who live there.

I make it a point to stop in to visit friends or relatives if only for a few minutes. Even the short stay is memorable for them and leaves you both with a pleasant feeling of the occasion. Fortunately, we planted a fruit orchard sixteen years ago when we built here on the hill. Now I take apricots, peaches, prunes, pears and apples, as each variety ripens, to my friends that have left the neighborhood for assisted living facilities or the local nursing home. I often go empty handed but it is fun to see the smiles on their faces when I present them each with their annual homegrown products.

I feel guilty when I return to the nursing home to find that John has had a problem while I have been away. Our eldest son, Mark, put my guilt aside by saying, "As long as Dad gets better again after a few days home, you need to get away occasionally." He is right. We are both better for it when I return refreshed.

Trying to plan for my own future, last summer before my sixty-fifth birthday, I purchased long-term care insurance that included either assisted living or a nursing home. By during this and being prepared for the future no one in the family will have to take care of me. When I mentioned to our daughter-in-law that I didn't expect anyone to do this for me, she asked why then was I doing it? I said, "Because John is my spouse." I felt that buying the insurance was necessary before I get a serious illness myself and become uninsurable to cover my own future. Maybe the old saying, forewarned is forearmed, will be true.

DAILY LIFE

Sharing my life with John can be both busy and interesting. John is still so active that it keeps me hopping just trying to keep ahead of him, both physically and mentally. I can understand why nursing homes get mobile patients up and dressed. I believe keeping mobile patients going gives them the feeling that they are still part of the living world when I am sure that they have days that seem like it would be easiest to just lie down and quit.

After I help pull John up and out of bed, I assist in dressing him while he is still sitting on the toilet. He will button his shirt after I start the top one so they will come out even. He will pull on his own socks. Sometimes just onto the toes, or other times all of the way up depending if he is just out of the shower and still a little damp, or if the socks are stretchy. He has quit putting on his socks since I started this book and it is a small thing but they are beginning to add up.

Putting on John's shirt or jacket at times can be a problem; he really does not try to help much. I have found that it is easiest if I can put both arms into the sleeve holes from the lower back at the same time, and then pull the garment up onto his shoulders. It can really become a job while he is sitting down so I usually wait until we are both standing.

John will hold up the front of his diaper, while I hook up the side tabs. He seems to understand that the pads are necessary. Luckily, he has never had a diaper rash. I use Vaseline on him if I feel there might be a problem coming on, such as a drying area on the skin that he feels the need to scratch. John will put bloody streaks on himself before he stops scratching, as Alzheimer's patients can become compulsive at times.

One of my biggest worries for John is an impacted bowel. I use a lot of fruit and roughage in his daily diet. If there is a question about his regularity, I will give him some natural fiber in his morning glass of juice. He drinks his juice with a spoon, as if its gelatin, because it thickens up faster than he can drink it. I have also tried a mixture of prunes, applesauce and bran that is stored in the refrigerator. If this mixture is given a couple of times a day, it will take care of irregularity. Nurses use this mixture in one of the nursing homes and call it p.a.b. for the three initials of the ingredients. They give it one or two spoonfuls or one or two times a day depending on each patient's personal needs.

If he goes to the other extreme and has diarrhea, I find it easiest to undress him while he is again sitting on the toilet. Then I let him wash himself in the shower, while I hold onto the sprayer hose outside the door. A dose of fiber again takes care of this problem. I do not know how it can work either way but it does.

John can still feed himself and especially likes breakfast cereal with fruit on it. He usually eats all the food on the far side of the dish or plate first. When I turn the container around, he will then eat the other half of the food. I have yet to figure out why he does this. I know that stroke victims will often eat one side vertically but John does it horizontally.

John seems to be afraid of hot food, so I reassure him it is just warm. I will feed him the first bite just to prove it. If I break bread or crackers into John's soup, it seems to help him keep the liquid on the spoon by absorbing and thickening it.

John will just look at, instead of eating, a spoonful of food that has anything hanging over the edge of it. You can imagine how long it takes him to eat spaghetti. I have to cut it into small pieces. I do not know if John is being neat or has forgotten that his mouth is as large as it is. He will just hold the over full spoon up in front of his mouth until I notice and knock off the offending piece than he will continue eating.

John will get up from his chair with a spoonful of liquid food such as dry cereal and milk and walk around. This makes for a very smeary floor, because on the next trip he will step into the mess and spread it even farther. Short of tying him into his chair, I have not solved this problem. I have tried barricading him off with other chairs, but he just moves them aside and walks off with his spoonful of food. I just recently took an old leather belt and threaded it through his wooden stool's back rungs. Then I belted it around his waist or just through his belt loops and I call it his seat belt. He has yet to walk off with the stool, so maybe it is going to work. Getting a chair that he is locked into seems a little drastic at this time, but they seem to be used successfully in nursing homes. The seat belt method is working for now and has even set up the pattern of staying seated even when I don't use it. He still seems to assume he is locked in the chair.

I try to keep snack food set out on the counter at his sitting area, so he can pick it up as he walks by throughout the day. Encouraging extra eating helps to keep his body weight where it should be for his height and age. Alzheimer's patients even in the early stage can have noticeable weight loss even if eating normal amounts of food. Research has indicated the weight loss might be caused by increased metabolism.

I cut up all food into bite-size pieces, as John hasn't used a knife for about three years. He can handle sandwiches easier if they are cut into five sticks across the width. I keep an antique spoon pot of silverware at his end of the counter to serve him, which saves steps for me. I slice carrots and wieners length-wise because of the fear he will choke. I avoid giving him large, round candies or large nuts. I try to use the same common sense that an adult uses when taking care of a child. John is inclined to eat anything that resembles food if he feels hungry and decides to cook for himself. He has even eaten potpourri and fruit shaped candles at other people's homes when it is his usual mealtime.

One time, while I was away at an appointment, John ate from a container of dead flies that was in our garage. The caregiver in charge rushed him to the hospital and the doctor decided to pump his stomach because of the chemical granules used to kill the flies. Only I knew that the chemical was several years old. I had put a small container in a barrel where I keep empty pop cans because the remaining drops of syrup in the bottom attract flies. I arrived at the hospital in time to see John lying on the emergency table looking at me with eyes, like a deer caught in headlights, as they pulled the hose out of his mouth. It was a frightening experience and one hopefully that will never be repeated. The entire happening made me feel guilty for taking out the pop cans that morning and not thinking about the fly container, for not being there when John needed me the most and for the stress it put on the caregiver. Thankfully, that is the only time that John has had to go to the hospital in all these years but I know that it will be inevitable that he will return in the future. It did make me all the more aware of his eating habits. I never had children or grandchildren, other than one who liked to eat dog food and dirt when young, consume the unusual things that John will, so I am not prepared for this as much as I should be perhaps.

Most days are not that unusual. Our daily routine is pretty basic and that is good for both of us. Alzheimer's patients are more securely comfortable with what they know and understand, as there is so much that is confusing or entirely lost to them already. John is busy all day walking out one door, around the deck and into the garage. Then he comes back into the house and out another door, stopping now and then to pick up a bite to eat.

Sexual changes are personal enough that I am not going to go into detail here, but some of you might be wondering how we handled this situation. Everyone, male or female, knows that a boy goes through various stages of interest in his new found attachment and proceeds through life with more or less desire depending on his own personality. In Alzheimer's Association study groups there was no indication that dementia patients purposely exhibit inappropriate sexual behavior. It seems to be only accidental self-exposure or aimless masturbation. They may undress because they need to go to the bathroom, or already have, or want to go to bed, or they just feel too hot.

John's sexual interests diminished through his life, right along with his other mental abilities. I can say from my own experience that the old saying of, "You don't know what you're missing 'till you lose it" is true.

HABITS

John never seemed to go through the hiding stage during which many Alzheimer's patients put things into places that they do not remember, then fuss because they think their belongings have been stolen. In nursing homes, a problem arises when patients move personal possessions from one room to another, meaning no harm. They may just think the object is pretty and shiny or theirs. Their short term memory is gone, but their long term memory may tell them they have owned something like it and the piece reminds them of their earlier life. Patients can wander from room to room feeling lost and have a need to seek the familiar.

John does pick articles up and will move them to another room, but always leaves them out somewhere in sight. The top of the clothes dryer is one of his favorite receiving areas. This would upset our daughter, Valerie, when she would have paperwork set out to read and he would trot off with it to his pile spot. I just felt we were fortunate he left things out where we could see them. I call the activity "mousing things away."

Silverware can be almost anywhere, since a lot of his eating is done on the move. He will fork a bite, walk around, eat the bite off the fork, and often set it in whichever room he is in at the moment. I remember John walking around Valerie's new rental home with a glass of water. I didn't think anymore about it until we got home and she called to tell me that Dad had set the full glass down right in the middle of her bed. I told her just to be glad that it wasn't grape juice.

I was told at the research center that patients often remember parts of their life that were important to them. They said a man who could do little else could still play pinochle. John was a fine mechanic all of his adult life on the farm, but he could not tell the difference between tools after he got Alzheimer's. If I would ask him to bring me a screwdriver, he would get a hammer or some other tool even in the very early stages, soon after diagnosis. When I worked in the yard I would try to get him to help by having him push a wheelbarrow or lift a rock. It was as if he was thinking, "No way. If you are that dumb, go ahead, but don't count on me." It would make me upset until I finally decided it was less irritating to us both if I would just do it myself and accept our situation. This was hard for me, as help would have been great. Maybe this is why some men hate to retire until they have to because of their age. John had a much bigger yard to keep on the farm then our house had and he always seemed to keep them separate in his mind.

It would be nice if John had something he liked to do for entertainment but he never had a hobby. A farmer does not have a lot of time to do extra activities. He and our sons did go hunting each year in the fall. I gave them John's guns in the very early stage to get them out of the house because I could no longer be sure what John would do with them.

We always followed the boys and their sport teams. It was pleasant to be able to go to a weekday football or basketball game or track meet. We always thought that was one of the main advantages of living on the farm. Then he would just catch up on his farm work on Sunday, when necessary and then the boys would help him and they were learning by doing. This came in very handy later on without anyone realizing it would ever become necessary so early.

In the first stages of the disease, John sat for hours and watched sports on television. He had never before shown any interest in doing this. I think it was something he knew other men did and felt it was a safe world for him to enter. He now had no demands being made on him or decisions to make for himself or others as he had earlier in order to run the farm efficiently.

Keeping busy helps people to maintain their abilities, independence and prevents depression, which often accompanies memory loss. My problem was trying to find something John wanted to do. Looking at old photo albums, watching videos of World War II or thumbing through books from the library with large colored pictures interested him for a while. We soon passed beyond that phase.

John always sits at a certain place at the kitchen counter, and no where else will do. I set his food treats, such as dried fruits or vegetable sticks, there all day because he knows they are there for him to eat. The main problem I have is remembering to never set anything there that I don't want him to eat, as he will try. He also has only one place that he will sit at the dining room table. If someone sits there unknowingly, John will stand there and stare at them until they get the message. We call him our Archie Bunker.

John also does what is termed as "fingering." When I put him to bed and cover him up, he will sometimes pull the sheet over the blankets and smooth them back and forth. If I give him a pile of peanuts, he will line them all up in a row on the counter. I thought he was doing these things because he had always been a very neat person but as I watched him I realized it is more like a compulsion. Sometimes he will rub his finger up and down his leg again and again. I can remember him rubbing his foot on my leg, when we were in bed, and almost rubbing a hole in it before I would move my leg many years ago. I still have to watch that he doesn't rub up and down his own bare legs to the point of irritation, while sitting on the toilet.

We are now trying to cure a pressure sore on John's heel that he got from agitated behavior while in bed when I left him one time in respite care. I discovered that he was crossing one ankle over the other and the nurse said bedsores could happen in just a matter of minutes. It is true when they say that the part you see is just the tip of the iceberg. John's had a slow healing process but I had to win that battle, as it was so sore he didn't want to step on his foot. He just wanted to stay in bed. The health nurse got us an absorbent, cover dressing called CombiDERM that I can highly recommend. When the dressing is left on the wound, it will wick out all of the inner infection slowly day by day. Now I am putting a foam boot on John's one foot anytime I lay him down. This is a preventative measure to cushion his ankle if he crosses one over the other as he sleeps. John is getting so used to it that he will lift his leg for me to slip it underneath.

Some patients see their reflection in mirrors or in the glass on pictures and are afraid that someone is about to attack them. Others will turn and go in the opposite direction or will think it is a visitor so they will stand and visit with their own reflection. The hallucinations a patient with dementia often has are a sensory experience (seeing, hearing, or feeling) which can't be verified by anyone else. Approximately one half of Alzheimer's patients experience this according to the association. It is best to reassure the patient during these times and not argue with them, as their reality is their truth.

I have read of good reports about the prescription of the drug Seroguel. You can start with 25mg. And work up to as high as 400mg. It will take a few days to work but suggest you ask your doctor about this new drug if your loved one is prone to hallucinations

John has been paranoid only once. We were between research drugs and had to clear out his system for a month. He was to take no medicine at all in order to get ready for the new drug and progress on to the next research program. He kept getting out of bed and going upstairs. When I asked him what the problem was, he explained, "There is someone up there." I took him upstairs and showed him the house was empty. When I asked him if he had heard someone walking above us, he said, "No, but I just know they are there." I told him of the drug change and explained to him that he was having what is termed paranoia. I said that everything was fine and he did not need to get out of bed again. He said, "Okay," and never did. I have been surprised at the faith and trust he has always shown towards me as his caregiver. I suppose it is like a child towards his mother.

SOLUTIONS

As a caregiver, I have had to figure out ways to outsmart John at times, in order to do things for him that he can no longer do for himself. When John was still able to go into the grocery store with me and I lost him, I could always find him in the fruit section eating a banana. I would just find one the same size and have the cashier weigh that one twice. If I had him push a cart, John always headed for the check out stand with just one item. He never was a shopper, so as far as he was concerned it was time to leave and take the car for another drive.

With John being a wanderer, it makes him possibly leaving always a worry while in other people's homes. I think I have found the solution to this problem. We never owned a metal screen door, so he does not know how to unlock the new, black, metal locks that most people now own. If there is not a screen door, I can still put a coat or towel over the handle of the door. The old saying, out of sight, out of mind, seems to be right in this case. I have tried putting a chair in front of the door but he will just move it aside and proceed outdoors. If a door has two locks, he doesn't remember enough to unlock them both in order to leave. I have a bell on the doorknob of each of our exterior doors so that I have a general idea of John's walking cycle.

I was concerned by one of the local nursing homes that had all of their Alzheimer rooms in the basement, which was accessible by an elevator. I asked them what was it that kept the patients from just pushing the button and leaving? They said there was not a single person in that wing who knew enough to do that. My thought was, "How sad this is," but I did use the concept of concealing the seatbelt release button later when my husband kept opening the door and getting out of the car. He still understood the concept of escape with the car door button but not the elevator.

John cannot express when he is thirsty or be able to get a drink for himself. I try to have water or juice available for him at all times at his eating place on the kitchen counter. The easiest way to give him fluid is when I put him on the toilet. I will automatically hand him a glass of water at that time. Sometimes he will drink it all and sometimes he will only take a sip and forget what he is supposed to do.

Very few of us drink the minimum six to eight cups of water daily. When John returns from a nursing home, he will have very little urine output the first day; it will be very strong smelling and sticky. The concentrated solution reflects inadequate fluid intake. A lack of fluid in the diet can cause irritation of the bladder so I try to keep him flushed out.

Paper napkins are a particular favorite of John's. He will put them in his mouth and chew on them for days. Consequently I never let him have one, as it is easier to just wipe his mouth for him. It was one of the first things he quit using correctly initially, leaving it sitting on the table for the entire meal. It was as if he had no idea what to do with a napkin. After marrying John and coming to live at the farm, I helped his mom cook during: lambing, shearing and harvest crews, as well as for the general hired men. I don't really remember ever putting napkins on the table. Evidently they were not important in John's life and thus easily forgotten.

I failed to mention this paper eating habit of John's one time when I left him for a couple of days at a respite care center. You can imagine what happened. They automatically put a napkin at his place setting. He ate his meal then chewed up his napkin. With his cheeks full of a napkin, that was the end of his eating for the next day. I returned and when they told me of the problem I asked them why they did not just remove it from his mouth? The two girls in their twenties, who were in charge, said they were afraid he would bite them; and besides he just kept pushing them away from him.

Approaching an Alzheimer patient's face from the front seems to frighten them. I usually reach around from the back of John's neck if I want to remove anything from his mouth, or even put something into it like a toothbrush. Often if he will not let me do something for him, I wait a few minutes and try again. John will usually have forgotten he was against the original idea and then he allows me to proceed. Even in the early stages, patients with Alzheimer's seem to avoid frontal approaches. John will accept things better if given to him from the side. He can be very defensive of most things coming right at his face, as if he is afraid of being attacked. This time I sat him on the bed, put an article in each hand, entered his mouth from the side with my finger and pulled the paper wad out immediately and easily. The two girls were surprised at how easy it was to accomplish.

I now leave a note with care hints for John when I take him anywhere. I tape it to his nightstand and hope someone will read it. One caregiver did, and told me she found if she put a cookie in each hand, she could do anything with him. We all have our weaknesses, and she had discovered John's. It is a much better solution than trying to force him into doing something he has decided he does not want to let happen. He is so much stronger than I am physically that I have learned patience. Luckily, he is good and easygoing, and not prone to throwing me against the wall. If that were happening, this story would be about life in a nursing home I am sure.

About eleven years into the disease, John had periods of not eating. I had read a person with Alzheimer's could forget how to chew or swallow, and this really concerned me. The first time it happened, I was afraid it meant a major deterioration in his health. He would put a bite of food in his cheek area and just hold it there like a squirrel with a nut. It seemed to satisfy him that he had a food source stockpiled and would eat nothing else.

After trying everything I could think of, I called the Alzheimer's Association in Portland for advice. They put the problem into their computer and could only come up with the same things that I had been trying. They suggested rubbing his throat and the back of his neck, or massaging his shoulders. He seemed to enjoy all the attention but none of the suggestions convinced him to decide to swallow. I also tried imitating the chewing process and explained what he was to do and how to do it, but to no avail. When I would try to put a spoon into his mouth, he would just clench his teeth tighter and refuse to open his mouth.

Out of desperation, I stocked in a supply of liquid protein supplement cans and prepared for a bleak future trying to keep him nourished. I bought a sports bottle with a heavy plastic straw. I put the straw between his teeth and lifted it up so it almost just poured into his mouth forcing him to swallow. When he began swallowing the liquid, he also did the same with his stored food. Then I started spooning in other food, and he chewed and swallowed it. It was as if he remembered he could do that process after all. It sometimes takes several days before he will again feed himself, but so far I have managed to solve the problem. Since this first refusal to swallow, his quitting eating event has happened about five other times over the last few years.

When John quit swallowing, there has always been someone in the family with a sore throat. All I can guess is that John has also acquired it and has no way of letting me know. Perhaps John's throat hurts if he swallows food, so he doesn't; then he forgets how to until the pattern is broken. The sooner I use the straw the less time it takes for him to regain the eating skills. As the disease progresses, it is taking me longer to bring him around each time. I know this is a major problem in the fetal stage when the ability to swallow is lost or forgotten.

Eventually liquids will be a problem and cause choking. When this happens I will buy a thickening powder to add to the fluid and make it a pudding like consistency. This prevents aspiration or the inhaling of food or liquid into the lungs, and helps to avoid pneumonia.

When the patient first starts to lose the ability to eat certain solid foods, it is possible to blend the food to a pureed texture. Sometimes just a small change such as oatmeal to cream of wheat makes the difference. Keeping their weight a little above the norm is important if at all possible. It has been said that we should all carry fifteen extra pounds because of the possibility of sickness. My reply to that is, "I can get double pneumonia!"

HEALTH

Keeping John physically healthy is important to me since there is nothing I can do for his dementia. The Alzheimer's patient gradually loses the ability to interpret and express what is happening to their body or mind, so the caregiver has to do this for them.

John could always keep a house full of people awake with his snoring. I could always nudge him to stop if it became too bothersome. Besides, I always felt that if he was snoring, he was home where he should be and I did not have to worry about where he was. My mom once gave me those words of wisdom. With the Alzheimer's progression, his snoring receded. I assumed it was because he was not working hard anymore, so he was not as tired as he used to be when farming. I guess that was not the entire answer. About a year ago he started snoring again and holding his breath at times. The research nurse says it is because all of the brain connections are not working right and is part of the deterioration. I am back to nudging him again, but for a more urgent reason, possibly sleep apnea. Having him sleep on two pillows and on his side has helped. When I hear him holding his breath, and then snorting as he gasps, I will lift his head and put a third pillow under it. I do not know if it is the additional height, or if it is arousing him, but often this makes him quit holding his breath. Unfortunately this doesn't always work so I just keep shaking him awake until he changes his breathing pattern. If this gets worse, I may look into a small oxygen device for him to wear at night. Getting him to keep it on his nose could be a new challenge. Since I have put John on Aricept, his bouts with sleep apnea and even loud snoring have slowed way down. Recently I had a real scare as John woke me up about five in the morning by breathing really loud and fast and he was moving his legs around. He usually lies on his back and doesn't move at all during the night. This is another reason for the waterbed's buoyancy as it helps to prevent bedsores due to inactivity. I quickly turned on the light and could see that his head was under one of his pillows and his arms were under the covers and he didn't know how to remove the pillow. He was soaking wet to the point of having dripping water all over his body. I imagine he was going to hyperventilate from all the fast heavy breathing and he had himself in a position that he couldn't change. It showed me again just how vulnerable he really is at this stage. I told our daughter about it and she suggested that I put two pillows into one king size pillow case to control them better and that is what I have done.

Recently we drove to Portland for another research program. They are testing Melatonin on people with Alzheimer's disease and their caregivers. The goal is to help the patients that are up in the night wandering, as they can't sleep because they have their days and nights mixed up. It is a natural part of the body's function to regulate sleep with light and this decline occurs with age and Melatonin helps to regulate this. One night during the test period, John slept so well that he didn't even snore, so I may use this product eventually to help him get a full night's rest.

Along with his other research drug, I give him niacin to help his blood flow to his brain. Both of John's parents, when they were in their eighties, were diagnosed with hardening of the arteries. Their doctors prescribed niacin, so I am doing the same thing. I am observing that both of these drugs lower his blood pressure and that could become a problem.

Alzheimer's research published news, about four years ago, that vitamin E had helped the effectiveness of another type of research drug, so I decided it could not hurt to give it to John. Within a week's time our son, Kent said, "I don't know what you are doing differently with Dad, but he seems more alert." Now vitamin E is in the news as the latest discovery of medical research to help dementia patients. I give it most of the credit for John's stable health and take it daily myself.

Vitamin B complex has been added to our daily regimen. Two years ago a friend of ours was informed by his doctor that it was the only available treatment for his dementia. I assume that is because a lack of B12 can lead to dementia symptoms and it is important that your body has a good supply of it. This is now John's daily source of niacin also.

The herbal professionals believe that ginkgo supplements will help with blood circulation possibly including those vessels affecting memory and mental functions. Anti-inflammatorys, such as ibuprofen, are also being touted as a preventative to help prevent brain swelling. Along with other anti-oxidants, Vitamin C is often taken daily along with fruit juices for defense against colds and flu. After reading about magnesium deficiencies possibly causing Alzheimer's, I have now added this to John's daily regimen. A plastic container with daily compartments helps to keep both of us on schedule with our pills. This is also convenient when we travel.

Women, by the age of ninety, will be thirteen percent more likely than men to acquire Alzheimer's disease. Because of this fact, I need to suggest the use of the hormone, Estrogen for postmenopausal women. We are seventy-two percent of the population over age eighty-five and estrogen has been researched to help prevent Alzheimer's disease in women if taken early enough.

As I mentioned earlier, water is critical. Since John cannot express his thirst, I automatically hand him a glass of water every time I put him on the toilet. He drinks water better from a sports type container, as he will suck from the straw longer. He will often take one sip of water from the glass then forget to raise it up for the next swallow. He sometimes has more fun chewing up the straw than drinking the water. Holding the water container also helps keep him occupied while sitting on the toilet. I often hand him a piece of fruit or another treat while he is there.

Japanese-Americans have 2.5 times the Alzheimer's rate of Japanese living in Japan. Research shows that a person's diet a few years prior to the development of Alzheimer's is a more important risk factor than his or her diet earlier in their life. Therefore, older people should carefully watch their intake of fat and calories. The American diet consisting of refined foods, high fat, meat and sugar is a high risk factor for many degenerative diseases.

I have read medical literature suspecting the possibility of a virus that can be in our system twenty years before the first symptoms of Alzheimer's disease appears. It sounds like we would be wise to lead a healthy life at every age.

Several years ago, John was getting blue hands and feet. Because I was afraid it was a circulation problem, I took him to his doctor. I was told that water was no longer effective enough to prevent dehydration. He said I was to give him Gatorade, lemonade, or dry package noodle soup. In two days the problem was solved. I do not know if it is the electrolytes, salt or sugar that is so effective but it works and I often put this into his drinking cup. I try to feed John a lot of fresh fruit and vegetables daily. They are not just easy food for him to carry around and eat, but a good source of minerals, vitamins and fiber.

An annual physical is a requirement of our research program and a good practice for everyone. The blood work up is vital to show the doctor and the patient or caregiver how the body is functioning and I like to keep a check on John's liver reaction to his drugs.

John had a pneumonia shot the first year it was available, which is supposed to be good for life. He also gets a flu shot each year. I am allergic to albumin so my doctor discourages me from getting the shot. I will have the flu and John won't, so the shot seems to be working. I did ask last year if the pneumonia shot was cultured in egg also and no one knew so they asked the lab people and luckily it wasn't, so I finally got that shot and feel a little safer.

Luckily for him, John comes from a long line of very healthy relatives on both his father and mother's sides. They are long lived and there are no other known genetic diseases among his relatives. When an Alzheimer's patient has several illnesses at one time, it is harder to care for them. I have read that the patient is often in the hospital with something unrelated when the family becomes suspicious for the first time about Alzheimer's. I mentioned earlier that they become masters of deception so maybe when their guard is down with illness, others can finally see their problem.

John's father, mother and two close friends died during his very early stages, and that added to his mental stress and no one has decided what effect that has yet. The medical profession is trying hard to find reasons for the disease. The cause will probably turn out to be a combination of factors. All we can do so far is to try to prevent it and than care for our affected loved one when it does occur.

RESPITE

Respite is when the caregiver places the patient with another caregiver or in a facility for just a matter of hours or days instead of months as in a nursing home situation.

Sometimes just a few hours can revitalize the caregiver enough to keep the loved one at home for a longer period. Without respite the caregiver can become more run down and depressed than the person they are caring for daily. I remember asking how caregivers in the care homes can manage with ten patients when I only have one. The answer was, "We go home at night and get away from the stress." Personal caregivers also need to get away occasionally. I have been neglectful about doing this myself but I am getting better and strongly encourage other people to do it if at all possible. We live in a small community and there is no respite facility available here. I have used one when in Portland, and have really enjoyed the art museums and lunch for a few hours.

Since John's diagnosis, caring people often ask how we are doing, and I appreciate their concern. I tell them we are doing fine, and we are. I feel very fortunate that John has maintained his health and vitality as well as he has. My goal has been to keep him from the fetal, or last stage, for as long as possible. I do feel the one-on-one daily care in his familiar home surroundings has helped to make his life more comfortable. It has, however, taken its toll on me even if I do not readily admit this.

When I had my heart attack, and while I was in the intensive care unit, our sons put John in the local Alzheimer's home after one day of changing diapers. This was our first experience with professional care. It worked out so well; I now use them once or twice a year. It is important to refuel my energies and experience some of the life that we can no longer lead together.

The last three summers I have gone to an Elderhostel intergenerational week with one of our grandchildren. This is an experience I can highly recommend as a great way for two generations to mesh. The first time was with our oldest granddaughter Jennifer, to Ashland, Oregon and the Shakespearean Festival as she has always been interested in Victorian costumes. The next summer was with Robert, our oldest grandson. We hiked the Olympic Rain forest in Washington and experienced the beauty of old growth trees. Jake, our next eldest, chose a camp near Yellowstone Park in the Teton Mountains, where we rock repelled, rode horses, and canoed. Yes, grandma had to get in shape for that one. Aaron chose to see the Olympic Rain forest as his cousin had done. Mazie will go with me next summer and I hope to go right on down the line with all nine grandchildren as long as any of them want to go.

I have had a woman from senior services in several

times over the last year and hope to find someone to stay with John for a few hours every other week. Then I can attend our local home extension meeting once a month, and have a little social time with some of my favorite neighbors. Sometimes I like to just meet a good friend for lunch.

Our two farmer sons, Scott and Kent, are usually available if I need them, so I can have a few hours away from home.

They let their dad ride around with them, which John loves to do. I try to ask them only occasionally, as I know how busy and full their lives are as farmers and family men with three children each. It is important to me that they sometimes do care for their dad so they will feel they are helping cope with our sad family situation. I do not want them to feel eventually that they should have, or could have done more for either their father or their mother. In other words, I do not want to hear about it later, when it is too late for regrets. Our two children in Portland are also very good with their dad and help me when we are there. I feel very lucky to have good family support from all of our relatives on both sides of the family.

A new awareness of my future opened for me on an overnight bus trip. I was rooming with a woman exactly my age, who had cared for her spouse for sixteen years. He had early onset Alzheimer's disease at exactly the same age as John and was still going strong after four more years in a nursing home. This was an awakening to the fact that all the wonderful sights I was putting off for the future I may never see. Unless I start doing things now, while I am physically able to enjoy them, I will miss a lot of memorable experiences. The adventures that I don't get to do I won't know about anyway, but for now I will start slowly chipping away at my list of dreams.

SPEECH

Sometimes, John acts as if he is hard of hearing, but I think that actually it is my fault for not getting his attention before I speak to him. Otherwise, he will only hear the last part of what has been said and can't figure out enough to make sense of it; so he will miss the entire thought. When the patient only hears part of a sentence, it confuses and then irritates them, as it would any of us. Have you ever noticed an adult kneeling down to look into the eyes of a child to get their complete attention? You may have to even touch an Alzheimer's patient to get them to look at you long enough for them to understand what you want to tell them. Be sure to use short, specific, familiar words and simple sentences. It is very important to give one direction or ask just one question at a time.

If an embarrassing incident occurs, do not berate the patient but try to remain calm and matter of fact, and remember that the person is not being deliberately aggravating. They are more likely to cooperate if you are gentle and firm than if you are irritated and impatient. I feel that I lost my patience several times dealing with John's bowel habits, until I learned to accept the fact that it was now part of our daily life. I knew I had better change, because he couldn't.

A mind with dementia can go into overload easily. A lot of praise and touching helps to prevent depression that is caused by the patient's lack of understanding due to their short term memory loss. Months after John had stopped conversing, he would see a newspaper and read the headlines out loud. I was surprised whenever this would happen. It reminded me of the old story of the non-speaking three-year-old who finally asked for the potatoes at supper as he was being passed by. The startled family asked why he had never spoken before and he said," I never needed to." I sometimes wonder if I have anticipated John's needs to the extent that it made him overly dependent on me as his caregiver.

We had an eighty-year-old neighbor, Leamon, who was diagnosed with Alzheimer's disease. He would ask me, "How's the boys?" I would very carefully explain how each of the three was doing in detail, thinking how nice it was that he was interested. After I would finish my story he would say, "How's the boys?" I would then say "They are fine," realizing that was really all he wanted to know.

Dementia patients often repeat themselves or even scream or yell. Fortunately, John has never been verbally annoying. One day he uttered the same guttural sound over and over. I decided to try distracting him a few times until he forgot he was doing it. John has never done anything like that again. My younger brother, Dick, used to push my buttons when we were young by repeating what I had just said, so I am not sure how patient I would be with verbal repetition.

Often during the day I have the radio on for John, because research reports that Alzheimer's patients enjoy music. It can uplift and overcome disability in a magical way. Many dementia sufferers remember lyrics and tunes after their language skills are lost. This was true for John.

As Alzheimer's disease spreads through the cerebral cortex, it begins to take away language. About three years ago, and probably a year after John's entire vocabulary had turned into, "Oh, Shit," and, "Nellie, God damn it," we were getting ready for Christmas. In the other room on the television, a drum and bugle corps played the instrumental version of Jingle Bells. I was standing behind John, as he stood and softly sang the first two lines of the song. I would not have believed it if I had not been there, but it made my holiday. So, I know first hand the magic that music can produce. Many of the senior centers and nursing homes encourage dancing and have musical entertainment, because of the fond memories it invokes.

Some patients project themselves into a visual situation so nursing homes try not to show violence on television shows as subject matter for viewing. The patients may become frightened and agitated because it is hard for them to decipher the imaginary world from their own in their delusional state. The homes try to show mainly light forms of entertainment. I do feel the mental stimulation and fun they receive from the cartoons, sitcoms with a laugh track, animal stories, musicals and comedies are a visual and verbal aid to many of the patients. I know first hand that it is for John. Old movies and especially westerns seem to hold a man's interest, as that is part of their long-term pleasant memory from their past. John seems to enjoy television at times. It is my hope also that the audiocassette we hear as we drive along helps John's listening skills. I am sure he has lost a lot of word understanding, but he still seems to recognize certain terms that I use in the course of our daily living. Maybe it is because I have reverted to more childlike terms for basic functions and they ring a bell from his past youth.

It would give me great pleasure to have John cussing me out again. I miss the sound of another human voice at times, and I leave the television on more than I would like to just for the company of it. I always thought the best use of television was in nursing homes, but I have begun to feel that most of the patients are not really watching. TV is on and they are there.

POSITIVE SIDE

John is a lot of company for me. I tell my married friends that I never have to listen to any back talk, and anything I say and do is just fine with him. He is a companion to go to the movies with; I never have to eat alone; and he gives me a reason to cook a healthy meal for us both. John always loved fast food, so that is often a treat when we are in town. We can eat in the car at our own leisure. He is very easily distracted by watching other people in a restaurant and slows down his eating concentration. We do go inside sometimes for a fun outing. If I have someone to help me with John it is very beneficial to me. If I am alone with John, it is difficult to get him to sit down or to get him back up again.

When we were coming home on Amtrak about a year ago, I took him into the dining car. I didn't think I was going to get him out of the booth again, because he was having such a good time. There were other hungry customers, however, waiting their turn. After a struggle to pull him out of our booth I decided we couldn't eat on the train anymore, and from then on I packed a lunch. The train no longer goes through our area and I really miss it, as this was an easy way to go through an icy gorge in the winter.

When we travel anywhere now, double absorbent pads are always used. On a different trip I learned to avoid taking him to the bathroom on the train. He was doing just fine until he decided he enjoyed the motion of the train while sitting on the toilet. He refused to move! I tried every trick I knew, but no way was he going to get off the toilet. The compartment was the size of a small closet. Even when I got up behind him and tried to push him off with my feet, another Kodak moment, he just put both of his hands and feet out and pushed against the framework. Whether I pulled from the front or pushed from the back, John was determined to stay right there and enjoy the ride. Finally another man came into the area and I asked him to ask John if he could use the facility. This technique usually worked at home for me, but this time it did not work for either of us. The passenger finally went to the canteen and brought back a big candy bar, and that did the trick. He must have had small children at home.

After spending 75 miles in the restroom, our stop was next. I had begun to imagine us coming home the next day on the reverse train, from wherever John eventually decided it was time to get up off his throne.

I was, however, writing about the positive times! It is only much later this situation was so funny. I now do not think of it in a negative way. It was an experience that taught me to accept and expect the unexpected at any time. It also showed me any situation could change at a moment's notice.

John enjoys watching the grandkids and I feel he finds them quite entertaining. They are very good with him. I find myself more understanding of other disabilities now, and know our grandchildren are learning compassion and understanding because of our situation. I have taken different grandkids with us on both car and train trips. They help me by watching out for grandpa in a number of ways and are a lot of company for me. We just visit and visit, as I said earlier, I do miss the sound of another person's voice.

John was always more openly affectionate than I was. Touching is important in anyone's life, and I really miss that. Now I initiate hugs almost with strangers and sometimes I just rub John's head or scratch his back, as that was always a favorite with him. He usually pushes me away when I approach him from the front for a hug, so again I sneak up on him from the side. The other day he actually squeezed me back and that was fun and encouraging. A while back, he reached over in bed and pulled the bedcovers up and around me as I often do for him. I feel he may not be exactly sure who I am, but he does love me and still appreciates my care.

STATISTICS

The national Association for Alzheimer's disease states that it is the fourth leading cause of death in the United States, following heart disease, cancer and stroke. Approximately five to seven per-cent of people over sixty-five has Alzheimer's disease and about twenty per-cent of the population over eighty will develop it. By age eighty-five, 45 per-cent of the elderly will develop Alzheimer's. At least 40 per-cent of the nursing home residents have Alzheimer's or related dementia conditions. Currently, four million Americans are diagnosed with Alzheimer's. That number means that one in ten of us over sixty-five will probably get the disease. It is predicted that by the year 2050, 14 million Americans will have Alzheimer's disease because of the aging baby boomer generation.

In the past, people sixty-five and older who were experiencing Alzheimer's like symptoms were thought to be experiencing premature symptoms of natural aging. The chance of acquiring the disease increases with age and since women are one and a half to three times more likely to have the disease than men it seems to me that it may coincide with their increased longevity but studies have shown otherwise. It also stated that those who live until age 92 without having Alzheimer's disease probably won't ever get it.

Dementia has been described as a group of symptoms characterized by a decline in intellectual functioning severe enough to interfere with a person's normal daily activities and social relationships.

As of this writing, conventional medicine offers no effective treatment for Alzheimer's other than medicine that will stabilize the disease for a period of time into a plateau type situation, if they are one of the lucky ones. Most of the research was being focused on the changes in the brain rather than potential effective therapies, both preventative and maintenance but this is quickly changing.

We are fortunate today that improved diagnostic skills are available. Alzheimer's is now a specific disease that can be identified with testing. Early diagnosis is critical in order to start on medications that will possibly slow the disease's progression. This also gives the patient and his family time to experience adventures that had always been just a dream or something that they had put off to do "someday". Early diagnosis also allows the patient to participate and plan his estate and family finances, which later on can be a source of comfort for all concerned.

Common behavioral symptoms, such as paranoia, delusions, depression, agitation, sleeplessness and anxiety can be eased or eliminated with the use of psychiatric medicines. These symptoms make it harder for the patient to function or for the caregiver to help them. With the right drugs the patient will feel better even though the Alzheimer's disease is not improved. Remember that the body's sensitivity to medication increases with normal aging and a dementia patient is even more vulnerable to complications.

National nutrition studies have demonstrated that elderly people, who take vitamin and mineral supplements or herbal remedies such as Ginkgo biloba extract, seem to experience better brain function. Through my own experience, I feel that Vitamins E and B Complex have played a big part in maintaining John's physical and mental health, slowing what seems to be his inevitable decline. I wish I had been supplementing John's diet with these vitamins years ago, even before his diagnosis. I now wonder if his Alzheimer's disease progression might have been slowed down even earlier through the use of them.

THE NET

Last year our writing teacher introduced us to the inner workings of the Internet and we went on line. He typed in "alzheimers.com," and there appeared all the possibilities for information that I have been looking for all of these years. Now that I am on the Internet myself I have really been able to learn a lot about everything that I am interested in. The Net has the latest updates about Alzheimer's disease as they happen and if you hear news topics mentioned on the television networks you could read a more complete report on the web. I recommend it for every household.

Just recently I found what I was looking for those many years ago. A community board on the {alzheimers. com} web pages where caregivers communicate with each other and share their problems and solutions.

The teacher had suggested that my personal story would be good resource material to put on the Net. I felt, at that time, that computers seem to be more for facts and figures, not so much for feelings. Even though I feel the Net is used primarily by a generation younger than the audience I am trying to help is, a lot of users probably have parents or grandparents afflicted, if not spouses. Many of them may one day become caregivers, so I might eventually try to get my experience on the Net. I could be on a chat line through E-mail and talk with other caregivers first hand.

Rereading this chapter makes me realize that I need to update it. After two years on the computer writing our story and learning the value of the Internet I have decided to try to reach caregivers by way of the net by logging on to {selfhelpbooksnow.com}. You can find many useful books covering a wide range of subjects and this will be one of them. My brand new e-mail address is {Nellie409@yahoo.com} I got it to help answer any questions you might have after reading my book because I would love to correspond with you or yours.

According to participants at the "Care of People with Alzheimer's Disease in the Next Millennium" conference held by the Alzheimer's Association's Ronald & Nancy Reagan Research Institute, people often turn to their computers first, even before doctors, for health information. With more than 100 million users worldwide, more people are turning to the Internet for information than ever before. The new national website is www.alz. org. Log on and become well informed. Remember, "knowledge is power!"

Our teacher has said since the first night that he does not want us to lose our own "voice." This happens by over correcting language or changing in any way the manner in which we express our own thoughts and feelings. I am sure that he is right. I was mainly writing this for our own family and future generations who may be interested in their past.

Our daughter, Valerie helped to edit this book but she was meaner than the teacher was with my great form and composition. After she got her doctorate, she corrected a lot of undergraduate's research technical papers. Mine will not pass for anything very important, but it has been interesting filling these white pages with the feelings I have never told anyone else.

John was such an intrinsic part of his family as son, brother, husband, father, and grandfather. Alzheimer's has affected not just us alone. As a lifetime member of this community, he was a friend and neighbor to many others throughout the county of Umatilla.

The disease attacks all walks of life. Medical research is studying nuns who have a lower percentage of dementia. Some feel it is because they are keeping their minds very active by reading and praying. I have a difficult time believing that theory. A man in our first research program was a nuclear physicist. He was so antagonistic about taking his pills that they made him leave the program. Maybe he was not as smart as I thought! John takes his pills as if they are candy and is still very manageable. I am now reading of the importance of taking a calcium channel-blocker to help protect against Alzheimer's and that is the research drug that John has been testing all these years. Maybe we just "lucked out" as John would say and happened to be in the right program at the right time. This is one of the reasons that I really recommend that any newly diagnosed patient immediately get into a research program if it is at all possible. They haven't found a cure yet but why not become one of the lucky ones that is selected to test for it? When they do decide which drug will work it will take years to test it and put it on the market for the average patient.

As farmers we have heard that chemicals are the culprits, but then I hear about a city homemaker with Alzheimer's who has never sprayed alfalfa fields or a cowherd for flies. Doctors have told me that those people who will not use an antiperspirant because of the aluminum ingredients do not realize that the medical field feels the disease causes the deposits of aluminum at autopsy itself. There is also the theory that aluminum might stimulate the manufacture of free radicals, or toxic particles, in the body. These free radicals accumulate in the brain, causing the patient to slowly lose control of his brain functions.

I called the Association recently and asked about their newest brochures on shadowing, wandering, incontinence, and bathing. They are so good and informative with practical information on how to handle various situations and problems as they arise. People who have been recently diagnosed will now have good news along with their bad news.

Use the materials that are available and ask for help. Another good source is ADEAR or Alzheimer's Disease Education and Referral Center. Their phone number is 1-800-438-4380. Remember you are not alone as a caregiver. Use not only resources for information, but also your county senior services and your friends and family.

When someone asks if they can help you, just say, "yes," and then tell them how. Don't be afraid to ask for help, so you can have some time away. A friend or relative also needs to spend one-on-one time with their afflicted loved one. It is not just to build memories for themselves, but to feel good about helping someone else and doing their share in a hard situation.

I keep hearing the words, "I don't think John knows me anymore" and they feel there is no reason to come for a visit. No one really knows what a dementia patient remembers and what he doesn't. I do know that I remember everyone yet, and all caregivers need support and love more than ever before. It is easy to want to remember people as they were, but I have always considered that the "chicken" way to do things. Good communication is not used often enough in some families. Do not let yours be one of them. If and when you need help, and we all do, say so. Don't be like that cow on the tee shirt with your four feet up in the air.

FAREWELL

Comparing crop statistics, discussing the weather, and a lot of story telling are all a big part of a farmer's life, and John loved all of these. Even early on, he could not be part of all that, and his lifetime friends soon found it uncomfortable to be around him. They just did not seem to know how to handle our new situation.

One friend, Jerry, who had a stroke while on the surgeon's table for heart repair, was very good about getting several other farmer friends together and taking John to meet them for lunch. In the first stage, Jerry did this several times until he finally admitted he was no longer comfortable taking him and felt really bad about having to stop. I told him not to let that concern him, as he had been the only one over the years who had even tried to see John. Being ill had made him see the other side of an ailment and gave him compassion, just as it has me. Some of us have to live one problem to understand another and that just seems to be a fact of life. This has been a sad time for all concerned, as life seems to be going on all around us while we are in limbo. I often feel that my life is on hold, while we wait for an unknown future.

Sometimes I am glad that John has a memory loss and doesn't know, hopefully, what it is that he is now missing in his life. He laughs and seems quite content just eating and sleeping and letting each day slip into the next.

Just the other day I told our youngest son, Kent, that I was going to put my book in the self-help section of the Internet. I told him that I was doing this in order to reach people that are concerned for their loved ones in possibly the fastest method. Kent said that maybe that would help to give our family a better understanding of why their dad had Alzheimer's disease in order to let us give support and information to others and maybe for the first time, give our situation a more positive aspect. Hopefully something good does come from everything bad.

The state of Oregon at this time has legal euthanasia and when the fetal stage becomes unbearable for John this would be one of our family's options. It would have to be considered very seriously the last six months of life but with Alzheimer's disease the medical profession has proven that there is no possible improvement at that point of the patient's life. I wouldn't even question what John would want for himself but now the law is such that he would have to verbalize his wishes and of course he hasn't been able to do that for years.

Nurses have advised me concerning inserting a feeding tube when John is fetal and his swallowing process has been forgotten. It was to not do it. I have recently read a report from John Hopkins medical center that decided tube feeding increases the rate of aspiration pneumonia and causes a variety of infections. They also state that a host of adverse effects accompany the use of tube feeding and two-thirds of the tubes will need replacing and the use of them should be carefully considered. Maybe it is our body's way of catching up physically with the mental deterioration of the advanced dementia patient.

The doctors have said the end for John will probably be a case of flu or pneumonia. I told them I did not understand that because his lungs are so strong and healthy. They explained that Alzheimer's Disease starts in the front of the brain and works progressively backwards destroying different vital functions as it advances, and ends up at the base of the head above the spine. That is where our immune system is controlled, and when it is destroyed we are left vulnerable to infection. Years ago when I questioned my favorite doctor about why people still died of pneumonia since the discovery of penicillin; he told me that pneumonia is an old person's friend. I have tried to hold on to that thought.

AUTOPSY

There is a nationwide network of more than two hundred chapters of the Alzheimer's Association. I can call the 800 number in Portland, Oregon, when I want tapes, books, pamphlets or just information off their computer. Anyone can call 1-800-272-3900 to the National Association in Chicago, Illinois to find their local chapter, if they do not already know where it is located. The Alzheimer's Association is the only voluntary national health organization dedicated to conquering this disease through research. It provides assistance to individuals with the disease and also their families and caregivers.

Work is underway to develop treatments and a prevention that would enable individuals to live dementia free for years, even after diagnosis. The medical profession eventually hopes to be able to treat individuals with a vaccine to prevent ever-acquiring Alzheimer's disease. In an effort to increase Congressional leaders' understanding of Alzheimer's and encourage discussion of policies related to the disease, Congress just this fall of 1999, has formed a bipartisan task force on Alzheimer's disease. They are hoping to better assist people with the disease and their families by working with the national association. The battle should soon be won!

Anyone diagnosed younger than age sixty-five is considered to have early onset Alzheimer's. John was afflicted with the disease at fifty-three years of age. Our four children and John's four sisters are concerned with their genetics, because their mother, at about age eighty-five, was suffering from dementia. We used to excuse unusual behavior with the typical saying of, "Oh, she is just getting old." I can remember her wandering down the street and in and out of stores, and when I would finally find her, she would wonder why I had been looking for her. She would laugh and say that she knew where she was. As John progressed into the disease, I remembered many times how his mom had acted in so many similar situations. Also, John's maternal grandmother had hardening of the arteries and delusions. I can remember her thinking there was a cougar under her chair and evil people outside the window attacking John and her being terribly afraid of what she was seeing.

John's dad always said he was afraid that his wife would, "End up the same way as her mother." He died before she did, and never witnessed the last years of her confusion, but he had been right in his fears. At that time no one in the family was experienced enough with Alzheimer's to know what we were living with or witnessing in grandma's situation. Now we know, and we fear for the future as research studies have identified potential genetic links. When definite links are found to be predictive, genetic testing may become widely available. The genetic linkage would be more likely in John's family if his mother and her mother had all had early onset, which they did not. They probably were just among that elderly fifty percentile.

Testing for Alzheimer's disease has progressed in the year of 1999. A urine test is now available for common diagnosis. Because there is no cure yet for Alzheimer's, the value of genetic testing still remains questionable. In some cases, having a gene associated with the disease does not mean a person has or will develop Alzheimer's. The national association recommends that, "Anyone considering a genetic test should do so in consultation with their physician and only with proper counseling." A positive test could cause unnecessary anxiety, anger, depression and stress. One of the biggest threats to individuals who undergo testing is related to privacy and possibly losing certain insurance privileges

One of the pamphlets I have is titled, *Autopsy-A Lasting Gift For Your Family*. It says that even though diagnosis has become more accurate in recent years, a brain autopsy is still the only way to prove that an individual has suffered from this disorder. There can be more than one dementia present, and an autopsy will prove which dementias are present. There is also a need for healthy brains to be donated for autopsy for comparison purposes. The autopsy is a lasting gift for your family, because it provides a vital record for the families medical history. Early onset Alzheimer's Disease represents only a small percentage of cases, but has been linked to several genes and runs through generations of families.

Individuals can make their own autopsy decision early in the disease or it can be made later by the spouse or eldest child as next of kin, if the spouse is deceased. If desired, families can choose an open casket as part of the funeral arrangements, since the brain autopsy will not be evident. Because the causes of Alzheimer's Disease are not known, the association recommends against donating any body organs for transplant purposes. Since John has participated in a research program through the course of his disease, that center may provide the autopsy. The next question is whether or not our family wishes to do this.

The newest demand is for unaffected brains to be used for comparison purposes. Anyone 55 or older can be a donor. A trained volunteer to ask questions about medical history, health and memory will call the donor once a year. Enrolled individuals will be given a special donor card to carry, and must sign forms in advance authorizing a brain autopsy when they die. Arrangements have been made for this service to be provided at no cost through your local donor program. Since I am the one that always carried a donor card, not John, I will have to keep my brain healthy.

EPILOGUE: FAMILY

Our four children have each understood and accepted their father's illness in a different way. Alzheimer's spouses also experience various types of willpower and stamina issues. No one should say that whatever we do is right or wrong until they have experienced something similar in their own lives. All we can do is the best we can for our loved ones and ourselves as we go on living daily.

I want to stress again the importance of visiting the elderly who are no longer able to get out and about. What goes round comes round is an old proverb and it is so true when it pertains to aging. It is to be hoped that most of us will live to see old age, so we need to be compassionate and understanding now to others. It is easy and inexpensive to send a note of cheer or to take someone a piece of fruit. Everything is welcome when given in love, but the best gift is a gift of yourself. John's mom, Gladys, always said, "We find time to do what we want to do in life." I often think of that when I hear people say they just cannot find the time. It often takes only minutes to do a little nicety for another. There is no time like the present.

"Nationally, more than sixty percent of nursing home

residents never have a visitor." This was printed in the Dear Abby newspaper column August, 1998 and was then a recent statistic. Abby stated, "The most effective cure for loneliness is caring, human contact". I have surprised myself and have become a hugger because I miss that contact and know others may also. And in that small way, we are helping each other.

Now that I am in my mid-sixties, I view the future through entirely different eyes. If I could have foreseen the future as a nineteen-year-old, and known that after thirty-three years of a very good marriage that John would get Alzheimer's Disease, I wouldn't have questioned whether or not to marry him. It would have seemed like a lifetime of happiness before anything adverse entered our lives. The trade off would have been accepted willingly.

In my maturity, I now know how fast the years pass by and how likely becoming a caregiver again would be if I should ever find a new partner at this advanced age. I really do not feel I could ever let caregiving become part of my life again. My life has been on hold for a large portion of it and enough is enough. I do not regret my past, but I will wisely plan my future. However, at this point my mom would say, "Never say never."

• • • •

Our older son, Mark, feels that keeping his dad on the family farm where he grew up helped him to feel content. The familiar sights that he loved and walked by daily gave him a feeling of purpose. Also family and friends were more comfortable going to the ranch for a good visit and to enjoy trips down memory lane while they still could.

Life in a nursing home would have been too confining for dad, we feel he lived longer in the home that he loved one on one.

Scott, our middle son:
"I had a great childhood. Dad was involved with fishing and hunting. We worked side by side on the farm, and he taught us everything I know. He never missed a sporting event that I played in, even if it was on a weekday, he would work Sundays to make up for it. He was always there for us."

Kent, our youngest son:
"Dad was a pleasant guy to be around and a great father. I couldn't ask for a better one."

www.ingramcontent.com/pod-product-compliance
Lightning Source LLC
Chambersburg PA
CBHW021112130626
46554CB00002B/661